PSYCHIATRIC RESEARCH IN PRACTICE

SEMINARS IN PSYCHIATRY

Series Editor
Milton Greenblatt, M.D.

Director, Neuropsychiatric Institute Hospital and Clinics

Professor and Executive Vice Chairman
Department of Psychiatry and Biobehavioral Sciences
University of California at Los Angeles
Los Angeles, California

Other Books in Series:

PSYCHIATRIC RESEARCH IN PRACTICE

BIOBEHAVIORAL THEMES

Edited by

E. A. Serafetinides, M.D., Ph.D.

Associate Chief of Staff for Research and Development
Brentwood Veterans Administration Medical Center
Professor of Psychiatry and the Biobehavioral Sciences
Neuropsychiatric Institute and the Brain Research Institute
University of California, School of Medicine
Los Angeles, California

GRUNE & STRATTON
A Subsidiary of Harcourt Brace Jovanovich, Publishers
New York   London   Toronto   Sydney   San Francisco

RC
337
P76

Library of Congress Cataloging in Publication Data
Main entry under title:

Psychiatric research in practice.

   (Seminars in psychiatry)
   Bibliography: p.
   Includes index.
   1. Psychiatric research.   2. Psychotherapy.
3. Psychobiology.   I. Serafetinides, E.A.
RC337.P76   616.89′0072   80-28012
ISBN 0-8089-1316-6

Grune & Stratton, Inc.
111 Fifth Avenue
New York, New York 10003

Distributed in the United Kingdom by
Academic Press Inc. (London) Ltd.
24/28 Oval Road, London NW 1

Library of Congress Catalog Number 80-28012
International Standard Book Number 0-8089-1316-6
Printed in the United States of America

Contents

Preface

The objective of this book is to examine how research affects practice—and conversely, how accepted practices may determine research directions in psychiatry and the biobehavioral sciences. Examples of current practices based on recent research contributions are discussed by various authors and compared where possible to existing empirical and nonresearch-derived practices. The implications and possible future applications of currently conducted research for therapeutic and preventive practice are also discussed, and the role of clinically generated needs in determining future research trends is considered.

The book is divided into four parts. Each has a particular theme or themes which bind together the respective contributions of that segment. Thus, "Old and New Themes" (e.g., schizophrenia and cytogenetics, cerebral dominance and psychopathology), "Practical and Theoretical Themes" (e.g., psychopharmacology and neuroendocrinology, as well as rationale for drug treatment), "Interactional Themes" (e.g., psychosomatic instances and psychotherapeutic applications) and finally "Complex and Ultimate Themes" (e.g., cultural and ethical issues) comprise the scope and range of the subjects explored in this way. Each segment is introduced authoritatively, but it is the purpose neither of the introduction nor of the expert individual contributions per se, let alone of the segments or of the book as a whole, to be all-inclusive. With the present flux of information we know that this is not possible. What this book does hope to offer to the reader through the use of selective landmarks is a stimulus and an opportunity to pause and ponder on the intriguing configuration of research and practice in psychiatry and the biobehavioral sciences. Anything beyond that, be it facts gained or ideas conceived, let alone actions generated, is pure bonus.

Finally, there is an underlying assumption, both in conceiving this book and in executing it, which ought to be spelled out clearly since it is (or it should be) of great importance in these times of societal and budgeting reconsiderations; namely, that research and practice are in effect a continuum, and that one cannot exist without the other. This is worth emphasizing, since any arbitrary divisions, usually initiated and perpetuated for administrative or professional reasons (e.g., basic versus applied research) tend to obscure the essential unity and interdependence of all scientific endeavor.

E. A. Serafetinides, M.D., Ph.D.

Contributors

Norman Q. Brill, M.D.
Continuing Medical Educator
Brentwood Veterans Administration Medical Center
and Professor Emeritus of Psychiatry
University of California
Los Angeles, California

Ching-Piao Chien, M.D.
Professor of Psychiatry
and Director, Innovative Ambulatory Care Services
Neuropsychiatric Institute
University of California
Los Angeles, California

Betty S. Deckard, Ph.D.
Research Geneticist
Brentwood Veterans Administration Medical Center
Los Angeles, California

Jared M. Diamond, Ph.D.
Professor of Physiology
University of California
Los Angeles, California

Barbara E. Ehrlich, Ph.D.
Postdoctoral Scholar
Department of Physiology
University of California
Los Angeles, California

Edward Geller, Ph.D.
Assistant Chief, Neurobiochemistry Research Laboratory
Brentwood Veterans Administration Medical Center
and Associate Professor of Psychiatry (Neurobiochemistry)
University of California
Los Angeles, California

Lawrence F. Gosenfeld, D.O.
Staff Psychiatrist
Brentwood Veterans Administration Medical Center
and Assistant Professor of Psychiatry
University of California
Los Angeles, California

Milton Greenblatt, M.D.
Director, Neuropsychiatric Institute Hospital and Clinics
and Professor and Executive Vice Chairman
Department of Psychiatry and Biobehavioral Sciences
University of California School of Medicine
Los Angeles, California

Donald S. Hiroto, Ph.D.
Staff Psychologist and Chief
Depression Research Laboratory
Brentwood Veterans Administration Medical Center
and Assistant Adjunct Professor of Psychology
University of California
Los Angeles, California

Richard L. Hough, Ph.D.
Chief, Health Services Research and Development Affiliation
Brentwood Veterans Administration Medical Center
and Associate Professor, School of Public Health
and Associate Professor, Neuropsychiatric Institute
University of California
Los Angeles, California

Marvin Karno, M.D.
Associate Professor of Psychiatry
Neuropsychiatric Institute
University of California
Los Angeles, California

Steven S. Matsuyama, Ph.D.
Research Geneticist
Brentwood Veterans Administration Medical Center
and Associate, Research Geneticist
Neuropsychiatric Institute
University of California
Los Angeles, California

Richard J. Metzner, M.D.
Assistant Clinical Professor of Psychiatry
Neuropsychiatric Institute
University of California
Los Angeles, California

Robert O. Pasnau, M.D.
Chief, Division of Adult Psychiatry
Neuropsychiatric Institute
and Professor of Psychiatry
University of California
Los Angeles, California

Stefanie Doyle Peters, Ph.D.
Psychology Intern
Neuropsychiatric Institute
University of California
Los Angeles, California

Kenneth S. Pope, Ph.D.
Director of Psychological Services
Gateways Hospital and Mental Health Center
Los Angeles, California

Fritz Redlich, M.D.
Associate Chief of Staff for Education
Brentwood Veterans Administration Medical Center
and Professor of Psychiatry and Biobehavioral Sciences
University of California
Los Angeles, California

F. David Rudnick, M.D.
Assistant Clinical Professor of Psychiatry
Neuropsychiatric Institute
University of California
Los Angeles, California

E. A. Serafetinides, M.D., Ph.D.
Associate Chief of Staff, Research and Development
Brentwood Veterans Administration Medical Center
and Professor of Psychiatry and Biobehavioral Sciences
Neuropsychiatric Institute
and Brain Research Institute
University of California
Los Angeles, California

Louis Jolyon West, M.D.
Professor and Chairman
Department of Psychiatry and Biobehavioral Sciences
and Director, Neuropsychiatric Institute
University of California
Los Angeles, California

Jeffery N. Wilkins, M.D.
Research Associate
Brentwood Veterans Administration Medical Center
and Assistant Professor of Psychiatry
Neuropsychiatric Institute
University of California
Los Angeles, California

William J. Winslade, Ph.D., J.D.
Co-Director, UCLA Program in Medicine, Law, and Human Values
Adjunct Professor of Law and Adjunct Associate Professor of Psychiatry
University of California
Los Angeles, California

Joel Yager, M.D.
Director, Residency Education
Neuropsychiatric Institute
and Brentwood Veterans Administration Medical Center
and Associate Professor of Psychiatry
Neuropsychiatric Institute
University of California
Los Angeles, California

PART I

Old and New Themes

Louis Jolyon West

Introduction

It is highly appropriate that Dr. E. A. Serafetinides should have been chosen to edit this volume on biobehavioral research contributions to psychiatric practice. The product of a classical university education in Athens, Serafetinides received the M.D. from the University of Athens. Following a medical internship at Athens City Hospital, he went on to pursue specialty training in Neurology and Psychiatry in Athens and London (both at the Maudsley and at Queen's Square). In England he also received training in psychoanalysis and in group dynamics (Tavistock). He went on to become an accomplished electroencephalographer and a clinical investigator, specializing in behavioral and clinical neurophysiology, receiving the Ph.D. from the University of London in 1964. The following year he joined the faculty at the University of Oklahoma School of Medicine, and soon won a five-year NIMH Research Career Development Award. In 1972, he took his present post as Associate Chief of Staff for Research at the VA Medical Center, Brentwood, from which base of clinical research operations he also serves as Professor of Psychiatry at the University of California at Los Angeles, as Attending Physician at the UCLA Neuropsychiatric Institute, and as a member of the UCLA Brain Research Institute.

In the winter of 1979, the faculty of the UCLA Department of Psychiatry and Biobehavioral Sciences undertook a special intramural conference, organized by Professor Milton Greenblatt, to consider the direction that the Department should take during the 1980s. Three major thrusts were identified as relating to the greatest needs for the profession during the coming decade: first, to emphasize clinical work concerned with the psychiatric and behav-

3

ioral problems of physically ill patients (including all aspects of liaison psychiatry in the general hospital); second, to strive for greater psychiatric contributions to formulation of public policy in spheres where our expertise is legitimately involved; and third, to stress prompt and vigorous application of research findings in the biobehavioral sciences to the practice of psychiatry and of medicine in general.

Thus it is highly appropriate that this new volume, directed toward the last of the three issues defined above, should have been assembled under the immediate editorship of Serafetinides, as part of a series of which Greenblatt is the general editor. This, the first segment, contains three chapters ranging from the traditional to the unusual.

The first concerns progress in cytogenetics. The importance of this discipline has only recently been sufficiently appreciated by psychiatry. Drs. Matsuyama and Deckard, active investigators in the field, offer a panoramic and heuristic survey of the rapidly changing scene in this exciting scientific discipline. The review ranges from an historical overview to specific techniques and clinical applications in psychiatry. The final section on psychiatric patients is indicative of the progress already made in some crucial areas. More progress is clearly to be expected.

In the second segment Dr. Karno, an experienced clinical psychiatrist with a long-standing interest in schizophrenia, identifies a triangular relationship, illness experience, treatment principles, and biobehavioral research findings, in selected aspects of schizophrenic disorders. As a starting point, Karno utilizes findings on CNS information processing and its defects in schizophrenia, and relates them to clinical findings on attention. Other research findings follow and these again are related back to clinical observations. In this way, Karno shows how research and practice should be a two-way street. In so doing, he also demonstrates the importance of contributions by astute clinicians, and indeed by patients themselves, which, together with laboratory investigations, are leading to an improved characterization of the psychological deficits in schizophrenia.

Finally, Serafetinides himself, as a long-time student of cerebral hemispheric functioning, discusses certain aspects of psychopathology and associated electrophysiological findings in terms of laterality and dominance. This is an area of very rapid growth over the last few years, a growth not unmixed with controversy. Although it is still early to translate many of these research findings into clinical practice, there is unmistaken interest in the potential of this line of investigation. Serafetinides characteristically advocates caution, and additional critical research, in pursuing this line of inquiry, even though it is a line in which he is himself a pioneer.

Steven S. Matsuyama

Betty S. Deckard

1

Application of Cytogenetic Methods to Psychiatry

Man has sought to explain the workings of the human mind and human behavior for centuries. There is a vast research literature on mental illness, especially schizophrenia, manic-depressive psychosis, and senile dementia suggesting that a tremendous effort has been made to understand these psychiatric problems. Nonetheless, the etiology of these disorders remains unexplained.

The purpose of this chapter is to acquaint the reader with the methods of cytogenetics and to explain how cytogenetics may help to elucidate the underlying genetic mechanisms involved in the mediation of mental illness.

Human cytogenetics is a relatively young field of investigation and is a hybrid discipline which utilizes the concepts and methods of genetics and cytology to investigate the relation between chromosomes and the inheritance of morphological, physiological, and behavioral traits. The rationale for using cytogenetics as a method for studying the factors involved in psychiatric disorders is based primarily on the large body of evidence which points toward the importance of genetic factors in many forms of mental deficiency as well as in certain psychopathological syndromes (e.g., schizophrenia, manic-depressive illness, senile dementia). Thus the study of chromosomes, on which are located the hereditary factors, may provide visible evidence for

The authors wish to thank Dr. Lissy F. Jarvik for helpful suggestions in the preparation of this manuscript.

In preparing this chapter, the authors were supported in part by the Medical Research Service of the Veterans Administration and USPHS grant AG00776.

5

genetic aberrations and may furnish new insights into the etiology and pathogenesis of human behavioral disorders. These genetic aberrations may be expressed as a variation from normal either in number or in the structure of the chromosomes. Before explaining the techniques used in cytogenetics, and their past, present, and possible future application of psychiatry, we would like to acquaint the reader with some of the important discoveries that led to the fusion of cytogenetics and psychiatry.

HISTORICAL OVERVIEW

In 1903, Walter S. Sutton,[1] in an article entitled "The Chromosomes in Heredity", advanced the hypothesis that the hereditary factors were carried by the chromosomes. Sutton fused facts and ideas from what were then two apparently unrelated fields of investigation, heredity and cytology, to form the foundation of a new research discipline, cytogenetics.

Since the appearance of Sutton's article, other investigators have provided ample evidence that the genes (hereditary factors) are located on the chromosomes and that it is the chromosomes which are transmitted from one generation to the next. Research investigations carried out with the fruitfly, *Drosophila melanogaster,* provided the initial evidence for the assignment of a specific gene, to a specific chromosome[2] as well as for the arrangement of the genes in a linear sequence along the chromosome.[3] Bridges,[4] who also worked with *D. melanogaster,* formulated the idea of a balanced chromosome determination of sex, contradicting the view that maleness was caused by the lack of a chromosome.

The application of these ideas to human genetics awaited the refining of appropriate techniques for use on human chromosomes. In 1956 Tjio and Levan[5] correctly identified the human diploid chromosome number as 46, with 22 pairs of autosomes and two sex chromosomes (XX in women and XY in men). There had been numerous prior attempts to ascertain the correct chromosome number in humans, dating back to 1891, when Hansemann[6] reported chromosome numbers of 18, 24, and more than 40. In 1912, von Winiwarter[7] investigated spermatogonial mitoses and counted 47 chromosomes. He concluded that in females there were 48 chromosomes, including two X chromosomes, while in males the number was 47 with only a single X chromosome. The presence of a small Y chromosome in males was reported by Painter in 1921.[8] In that same paper he reported chromosome counts in the range of 45−48 but in the clearest metaphase plates he could find only 46; however, he was still uncertain whether the correct number was 46 or 48. Two years later,[9] working with testicular biopsy material from mental defectives, he concluded that the correct number was 48 (in retrospect, it may have been that these subjects were aneuploid). From that time on, until 1956, the human diploid chromosome number was accepted as 48. These studies were all carried out on sectioned material and large numbers of analyzable cells were not readily available. Thus, the large number of chromosomes, the wide range of sizes, and the tendency for chromosomes to clump, presented a formidable problem to ascertaining the correct chromosome number. (For a more detailed account of the controversy surrounding the human diploid chromosome number, see Ref. 10.)

In 1956 Tjio and Levan,[5] utilizing modern cell culture techniques and adapting older techniques (hypotonic treatment and colchicine) surprised the scientific community by reporting that the human diploid chromosome complement was 46 with 22 pairs of autosomes and one pair of sex chromosomes. The very high quality of their preparations made the possibility of error quite small and signaled the beginning of a new field, human cytogenetics. The chromosome number of 46 was rapidly confirmed by other investigators working with a variety of human tissues.[11,12]

In 1959, Lejeune, Turpin, and Gautier[13] reported that patients with Down syndrome (formerly called mongolism) had 47 chromosomes. The extra one is a small acrocentric chromosome designated as number 21, hence the other name for this syndrome, Trisomy 21 (47, XX or XY, +21). Confirmation of the chromosomal anomaly associated with Down syndrome quickly followed from a number of other laboratories[14,15] and provided the first evidence of an association between a specific chromosome abnormality and mental deficiency. In the same year several sex chromosome abnormalities were identified: Turner syndrome (45, X), Klinefelter syndrome (47, XXY) and the triple-X chromosome complement (47, XXX).[16-19]

The next nine years were characterized by a voluminous increase in cytogenetic data with contributions primarily in areas describing numerical and structural aberrations. No doubt the tremendous influx of data was the result of another breakthrough, the publication by Hungerford and associates[20] in 1959 of a method to culture human peripheral blood leukocytes for chromosome analysis. However, chromosome studies were severely limited by the inability to distinguish chromosomes that were morphologically similar, thus precluding precise identification of chromosomes. Further, structural rearrangements which did not alter chromosome morphology, such as inversions, went undetected. The technique of autoradiography, introduced by German,[21] proved helpful in identifying some of the chromosomes, most notably the inactive X chromosome. However, not all chromosomes could be precisely identified. Further, this method is tedious and time consuming and does not readily lend itself to routine use in the laboratory.

Then in 1968, another breakthrough occurred with the report by Caspersson et al.[22] that animal and plant chromosomes stained with the fluorescent dye quinacrine mustard and viewed under a fluorescent microscope, showed differential quantities of the fluorochrome bound to specific regions of the chromosomes. In addition, the fluorescent pattern along the length of the chromosome was consistent for homologous pairs of chromosomes. This initial report was quickly followed by a series of papers from the same group applying the fluorescent technique to human chromosomes.[23,24] Again, as found in plant and animal chromosomes, the fluorescence pattern was unique for each chromosome pair. These distinctive areas of fluorescence, known as Q bands, allowed for a more exact identification of chromosomes and their abnormalities than had been possible previously. At the molecular level, the intensity of fluorescence is a reflection of the base composition of the DNA; DNA rich in thymine and adenine enhances quinacrine fluorescence, while DNA rich in cytosine and guanine quenches fluorescence.[25,26] It was impossible, however, for all laboratories to engage in this type of research because of the expense of the fluorescence equipment.

Another technique to identify chromosomes soon became available and eliminated the need for fluorescence. This method developed from the observation that during in situ DNA/RNA hybridization experiments, the centromeric region stained very darkly with Giemsa, whereas the rest of the chromosome remained light.[27] Applying the denaturation reannealing technique to human chromosomes, Arrighi and Hsu[28] showed that all chromosomes were darkly stained at the centromere region and that certain chromosomes had larger stained sections than others. These researchers also observed darkly stained regions around the secondary constrictions on the long arm of chromosomes 1 and 16, and possibly 9, and also the distal half of the Y chromosome. These Giemsa stained areas are referred to as C bands. In the course of their staining procedure, these investigators noticed that chromosomes in metaphase spreads occasionally showed a pattern of bands similar to that produced by quinacrine staining. In order to achieve consistent banding, the centromere staining procedure was modified in a variety of ways. One such method was the acetic/saline/Giemsa (ASG) method,[29] which produced bands very similar to those resulting from the quinacrine fluorescence technique. These types of bands are called G bands. Other variations included: soaking in various salt solutions at different temperatures and for various periods of time; denaturation and reannealing at different times and temperatures; enzymatic treatment with proteases, the most common one being trypsin; and a combination of these various techniques. That these staining techniques were not readily replicable from one laboratory to another was evident by the plethora of new staining techniques which appeared in the literature, primarily minor modifications of previously published methods. There is even a technique to produce bands in reverse contrast to those obtained with quinacrine and Giemsa staining techniques.[30] These reverse bands are called R bands.

To improve communication among investigators, a uniform system of chromosome identification utilizing the banding patterns was proposed in 1971.[31] The basis for the identification of each and every chromosome was the band pattern obtained by quinacrine staining. The various techniques producing bands were abbreviated as follows:

Q bands = from quinacrine staining methods
C bands = from constitutive heterochromatin methods
G bands = from Giemsa staining methods
R bands = from reverse staining Giemsa methods

Since the development of these staining techniques, a variety of further modifications, uses, and elaborations have appeared in the literature. Using the quinacrine fluorescent technique, Pearson and Bobrow[32] showed that it is the short arm of the Y chromosome which pairs with the X chromosome during meiosis. Another group of studies, also using the fluorescent banding method, provide evidence that certain types of cancer may be due, at least in part, to abnormal changes such as translocations, insertions and deletions in the chromosomes of somatic cells.[33-36] Finally, because human chromosomes can be identified by their fluorescent banding pattern, it is possible to recognize them in somatic cell hybrid lines (mouse or hamster with human). Using different types of hybrid lines it became possible to assign certain genetic loci to specific human chromosomes.

The above modifications and uses of the various staining procedures, although they are very important, represent just the beginning of what can be accomplished with these new techniques.

Recent progress in cytogenetics, aside from its major role in clinical genetics, has led to a refining of the banding techniques to increase the number of bands that can be visually recognized. In 1971 there was a total of 322 bands per haploid set of chromosomes and by 1975 the number had risen to 923. This increase in the number of visible bands was due primarily to the use of late prophase preparations and the realization that some of the major bands seen at metaphase were due to the coalescing of many minor bands. A cell synchronization procedure recently introduced by Yunis[37] consistently gave a large number of cells in the appropriate stage of mitosis which upon staining produce 1256 bands per haploid set. Briefly, this procedure utilizes amethopterin, an agent which interferes with de novo thymidine synthesis, thus producing a nutritional requirement for thymidine. Upon release from this block, a synchronous burst of mitoses occurs allowing for the accumulation of metaphase cells appropriate for staining and analysis. This method has been modified by adding actinomycin D to the cultures prior to harvesting to inhibit the chromosome condensation process, and it is now possible to visualize a total of 1400 bands.[37a] Thus, human cytogenetics has entered into the high resolution stage and is beginning to bridge the gap between genes and chromosomes.

TECHNIQUES

Cytogenetic investigation requires that cells undergo division since chromosomes suitable for study are available only during the late prophase and metaphase stages of mitosis. Mitotic cells can be obtained directly from rapidly-dividing tissues in the body (e.g., bone marrow or germinal epithelium) or from tissue stimulated to divide in culture (e.g., peripheral leukocytes). Prior to 1959, a tissue biopsy was necessary for chromosome studies. With the advent of the human peripheral blood leukocyte culture system for chromosome analysis, the in vitro culturing of lymphocytes has become the most extensively utilized culture technique in chromosome studies. Very briefly, this method is as follows: Blood is drawn by venipuncture and placed in vials containing heparin. Then the leukocyte-rich plasma, which has been separated from red blood cells, is added to growth medium and incubated for two to three days. During the last hour of the incubation period colcemid is added to prevent spindle formation and to collect cells at the metaphase stage of mitosis. The cells are then harvested, treated with a hypotonic solution and fixed. The cell suspensions are used to prepare microscope slides which are subsequently stained.

These preparations are then ready for microscopic examination. In the routine method of examination, the slides are scanned under low power (125×) and metaphase cells which appear suitable for analysis are examined under oil immersion (1250×). Morphologically, these spreads should be round with few, if any, chromosome overlaps. The chromosomes in each cell are then counted and analyzed for abnormalities. For a representative number of cells, photographs are taken and from photographs the chromosomes are arranged in pairs in what is termed a karyotype. In the normal human complement there are 46 chromosomes, 22 pairs of autosomes and 2 sex chromosomes (XX in females and XY in males). The autosomes are serially numbered from 1 to 22, in descending order of length with special attention paid to centromere position, and are also divided into seven easily distinguishable groups (A through G).

For preparations which have been stained so that banding patterns are evident, the examination is much the same. As in the routine method, slides are scanned under low power and well spread metaphase cells exhibiting discrete banding patterns on the chromosomes are selected for examination under oil immersion. A photomicrograph is taken and a karyotype constructed, using as a reference the diagrammatic representation of chromosome bands agreed to by cytogeneticists at the Paris Conference.[31] While analyses can be carried out directly at the microscope, it is extremely tedious and for Q bands this examination must be done rapidly since the fluorescence diminishes very quickly. By a careful analysis of the banding patterns, structural rearrangements (e.g., reciprocal translocations) which do not alter chromosome morphology can be relatively easily delineated and if numbers greater or less than the normal number are present, the specific chromosome involved can be identified.

A companion technique to chromosome analysis is the sex chromatin technique (sex chromatin is also referred to as a Barr Body[38]). The sex chromatin number allows one to rapidly determine the number of X chromosomes in the complement, the maximum number of sex chromatin masses in the interphase nuclei being one less than the total number of X chromosomes. This technique is relatively simple and is used in population screening studies for assessing the frequencies of X chromosome abnormalities. It is used as a diagnostic aid when errors of sexual development occur and when sex chromosome abnormalities are suspected and is routinely used in screening women athletes at the Olympic games. Briefly, an epithelial cell preparation is made by gently scraping the buccal mucosa with a metal spatula and spreading these cells on microscope slides. The slides are then rapidly fixed, hydrated, and stained (a variety of stains can be used). The stained preparations are observed with oil immersion optics and the cell nuclei are examined for the presence of a darkly staining chromatin body positioned at the nuclear membrane. The number of cells containing sex chromatin is recorded with special attention to ascertaining nuclei with more than one sex chromatin mass. The prime error in this technique comes from buccal smears that are of inferior technical quality and can lead to an erroneous conclusion of chromatin negative, i.e., without a dark staining chromatin body, when it should be positive.

Since the advent of quinacrine staining and the demonstration that the distal half of the Y chromosome fluoresces very brightly, it has been possible to screen buccal smear preparations for the presence of a Y chromosome as well. This has been used in population screening to detect individuals with the XYY chromosome complement.[32] The limitations of this method are basically the same as those of the Barr body technique.

APPLICATION TO PSYCHIATRY

It is now well established that genetic abnormalities can interfere with intellectual development. The concept of ''inborn errors of metabolism'' was proposed by Garrod.[39] This is a genetically determined biochemical disorder, in which a specific enzyme defect produces a block in a metabolic pathway that may have pathological consequences. The first investigation of a biochemical defect, as a cause of mental retardation, began with the discovery of phenylketonuria (PKU) by Fölling.[40] He postulated that PKU was inherited and that the biochemical anomaly associated with phenylalanine metabolism caused the mental retardation. In subsequent studies[41-44] PKU was shown to be inherited as an autosomal recessive, and the biochemical abnormality was found to involve the enzyme phenylalanine hydroxylase, which converts the essential amino acid phenylalanine to tyrosine.[43,45,46] Although the nature of the link between this biochemical abnormality and mental retardation is as yet unknown, this work has provided a conceptual model for relating genes to phenotypes. Genes do not express themselves directly as behavior; rather, their effects are mediated through metabolic pathways, and a metabolic disturbance can cause behavioral consequences. There is much evidence which suggests that psychiatric disorders are determined, at least in part, by genetic factors. This evidence is especially convincing in the case of schizophrenia[47-51] and manic-depressive psychosis.[52-54] There is, as yet, no definitive answer to the question of how these disorders are transmitted from one generation to the next. The problem may be due, at least in part, to the fact that it is very difficult to rigidly define the various types of mental illness. For example, the diagnosis of schizophrenia subsumes different subtypes, a multitude of behaviors, and in addition, is dependent on the individual making the evaluation. Thus, the heterogeneity seen in psychopathologies may be due to defects at different steps in a common metabolic pathway. The study of chromosomes may help to explain the underlying genetic and biochemical mechanisms involved in mental illness, but so far has not provided any new insights.

Numerous chromosomal abnormalities are known but those involving the sex chromosomes are the most frequent (0.25% of all newborns[55]). Sex chromosome abnormalities are of interest to investigators in the behavioral sciences even when they occur without accompanying mental deficiency since they may have profound influences on psychosexual development and some of them have also been implicated in psychopathology. By contrast, the autosomal anomalies generally result in severe mental retardation so that it becomes difficult to separate the mental impairment from mental illness. It is for this reason that the following discussion is limited to sex chromosome abnormalities.

Sex Chromosome Anomalies

TURNER SYNDROME (45, X)

In general, these individuals are phenotypically female, with a chromosome complement 45, X (ie., there is only a single chromosome, instead of the expected two X chromosomes, and no sex chromatin body).

Although the most prevalent form of Turner syndrome is 45, X, there are about 30 percent of individuals with this syndrome who are sex chromatin positive, resulting from mosaicism (e.g., 45X/46XX) or an X chromosome structural abnormality.[56] There are also cases of "male Turner" individuals resulting from mosaicism (e.g., 45X/46XY/47XXY and 45X/46XX/ 47XXY.)[57-59]

Affected individuals are characterized by various physical stigmata including short stature, webbed neck, shield chest, low hairline, skeletal abnormalities, and cardiac abnormalities. However, the only consistent abnormality is gonadal dysgenesis, that is, "streak gonads" and sexual infantilism.[60]

The incidence of this abnormality is about 0.04 percent of female births.[61] Since these individuals are sterile, they are not able to transmit the disorder to offspring. However, there is some evidence from pedigree studies for a familial predisposition in certain cases.[56] There is no association between Turner syndrome and advanced maternal age. The frequency of this syndrome is not greater among institutionalized mental defectives than it is among the general population.[62]

Mental retardation is not a necessary concomitant of Turner syndrome; in fact, all levels of intellectual functioning are found in these individuals.[62,63] However, among these patients, there is a specific cognitive defect, *space-form blindness*,[64] which includes severe deficits on tasks that require right-left orientation. Further, these individuals perform more poorly on spatial, perceptual, and arithmetic tests than on verbal tests.[63,65,66]

The abilities most impaired in Turner patients are those that are more highly developed in males than in females, with a performance hierarchy progressing from best in normal males to worst in Turner patients (with normal females in between). Investigators have attempted to delineate the genetic component of spatial ability and the data are suggestive of a sex-linked factor.[67-69] Three studies of spatial performance have found a unique pattern of family correlations with unlike sex parent-child pairs (i.e., father-daughter and mother-son) exhibiting a higher correlation on test scores than like sex parent−child pairs (i.e., father−son and mother−daughter). These results are compatible with sex-linked recessive mode of inheritance for spatial ability.

Despite having a single X chromosome, the gender identification of these individuals is generally female, although they do not develop female secondary sexual characteristics. With regard to psychosexual development, Turner individuals exhibit no greater incidence of psychiatric disorders or homosexual orientation than the general population.[70] Since most are phenotypically females, they are brought up as girls and are feminine. However, during adolescence, they tend to be concerned with their physical appearance and those girls most delayed in physical development tend to be more emotionally immature.[70]

KLINEFELTER SYNDROME (47, XXY)

These individuals are phenotypic males and have a chromosome constitution of 47, XXY (i.e., they have an extra sex chromosome). The buccal smear is chromatin positive with a single Barr body. Other chromosomal variants subsumed under the rubric of Klinefelter syndrome have been reported, consisting of as many as five extra X chromosomes, extra Y chromosomes, various combinations of extra sex chromosomes, as well as numerous mosaics. The presence of the Y chromosome, regardless of the number of X chromosomes, leads to phenotypic maleness.

The clinical features associated with this syndrome include tall stature with long limbs, seminiferous tubular dysgenesis with sterility, small testes with otherwise apparently normal external genitalia, and sometimes gynecomastia. In general, it is in adolescence and young adult life that this syndrome becomes evident, at which time the inadequate sexual development or gynecomastia prompts the individual to seek medical consultation. Yet others show normal physical development and are discovered only when they present themselves at infertility clinics.

The incidence of Klinefelter syndrome is about 0.2 percent among newborn males.[61] Because Klinefelter males are sterile, there is no transmission of the anomaly from one generation to the next. Unlike Turner syndrome, there is no evidence for a familial predisposition to nondisjunction in this case.[56]

Mental retardation is not a necessary feature of this syndrome. There may, however,be some degree of mental deficiency and generally, intellectual attainment is below that of their siblings.[61] Hamerton,[56] in a survey of 22 studies of sex chromatin positive males, found that the incidence of mental retardation was three to five times the expected frequency of mental retardation in the general male population. With regard to the chromosomal variants of Klinefelter syndrome, the addition of an extra X chromosome appears to be associated with a greater degree of mental subnormality while an extra Y chromosome is associated with tall stature. (Additional discussion of the clinical manifestations of extra X and Y chromosomes can be found in the sections of the triple-X syndrome and the XYY syndromes, below.)

Persons with Klinefelter syndrome exhibit a higher than average incidence of psychiatric disorders, in many cases with the diagnosis of schizophrenia. Further, these patients often exhibit antisocial and criminal behavior, but not, however, to the same extent as patients with an extra Y chromosome.[62] This type of psychopathology may be due to a nonspecific effect of extra chromosomal material such that an imbalance results between the X and Y chromosomes. In terms of psychosexual development, many of these individuals suffer serious problems. Further, there is evidence which suggests that Klinefelter patients suffer varying degrees of gender reversal more often than expected by chance.[71]

XYY SYNDROME (47, XYY)

This syndrome is the most controversial of the chromosomal disorders. Affected individuals are males with an extra Y chromosome and a chromosomal complement of 47, XYY. This sex chromosome complement was first described in 1961[72] in a normal male and was followed by a number of isolated case reports. Many of the first investigators of the XYY syndrome observed a variety of associated physical stigmata, primarily hypogonadism[73]; however, in the majority of cases published subsequently there appear to have been normal sexual development.

Then, in 1965, Jacobs and coworkers[74] noted among prisoners who had been institutionalized for "dangerous, violent or criminal propensities" a very high frequency of individuals with an extra Y chromosome. Seven of 197 prisoners (3.6%) were found to have the XYY chromosome constitution and these individuals were also quite tall, their average height being 73.1 inches. If, in this sample, only those over six feet tall were considered, the frequency would be nearly 50 percent. Great height, borderline intelligence and aggressive behavior were the outstanding features of the XYY individuals. No other physical stigmata would differentiate them from other males. The XYY syndrome represents the first time a specific behavioral abnormality other than mental deficiency has been linked to a chromosome abnormality.

Since the original study by Jacobs et al.,[74] there have been many other studies of the behavioral manifestations of the 47, XYY syndrome. These reports generally confirm that an extra Y chromosome is associated with greater than average height, violent and aggressive behavior, and borderline intelligence. In a review of the world literature[75] the frequency of XYY individuals was compared among different male population groups (newborn, normal adults, juvenile delinquents, mentally ill males, and criminals). Further, the 47 XXY complement was used as a comparison group because some authors maintain that criminal aggressive behavior is as frequent in these individuals as it is in 47, XYY individuals. Among the newborn, normal adults and mentally ill males, the frequencies of XXY individuals were similar to that of XYY. Only among juvenile delinquents and criminals was the frequency of males with an extra Y chromosome significantly greater than that of the extra X chromosome. Similar findings have been reported by Hook,[76] who independently surveyed the world literature.

It should be noted that the studies reviewed have usually selected tall, violent prison inmates and other institutionalized subjects, which points to a sampling bias. While not all individuals with an extra Y chromosome will be excessively tall, nor display aggressive or antisocial behavior nor borderline intelligence, there is sufficient association for the triad so that it cannot be ignored. Prospective studies to assess the roles of heredity and environment are currently being carried out.[77-79] These studies are following the development of XYY males who have been identified at birth.

The incidnece of the extra Y syndrome is about 0.1 to 0.2 percent among newborn males.[75,76] There appears to be neither a maternal age effect[80] nor a paternal age effect.[73] There is scant information available about the fertility of XYY males since most of the reported cases were institutionalized and unmarried. It appears from the available data, however, that fertility is unimpaired. It is interesting to note that except for two reports[81,82] of 47 XYY offspring fathered by 47, XYY males, all children examined were found to have a normal chromosome complement.[72,83] The report by Diario and Glass[84] that 5 percent of the sperm from an XYY male has two Y chromosomes (as detected by the fluorescent technique) suggests that only a minority of sperm carry two Y chromosomes, and probably accounts for the low transmission rates. Chandley and coworkers[85] found normal meiosis in two 47, XYY males but found no evidence for the occurrence of two Y chromosomes in the germ line.

TRIPLE-X SYNDROME (47, XXX)

These females, although having an extra X chromosome, generally exhibit no major congenital malformations. They are sexually normal, that is, they develop female secondary sexual characteristics, are fertile and reproduce, although menstrual irregularities and early menopause may occur in some cases.[60]

The frequency of this syndrome among newborn females is about 0.1 percent.[62] Unlike Turner females, these triple-X females are not sterile and have reproduced. There are in the literature reports of 13 triple-X females who produced 12 female and 23 male children, all of whom had normal sex chromatin.[62] Statistically speaking this is a surprising finding since one would expect half of the offspring to have an extra sex chromosome, either XXY or XXX. Hamerton[56] suggests that there is some sort of directional selection during oogenesis such that the abnormal chromosome complement is included in one of the polar bodies.

The frequency of triple-X patients in institutions for mental defectives is about 0.37 percent,[60] which is significantly higher than that for the general population. In general, the greater the number of extra X chromosomes, the greater the frequency and degree of intellectual impairment; however, there are individuals with the XXX karyotype who exhibit normal intelligence.

There is also an increased frequency of triple-X patients with psychiatric problems, generally diagnosed as schizophrenia or paraphrenia.[62] Both the mental illness and mental retardation could represent a nonspecific effect of excess chromosomal material. It is as yet unknown whether the extra X chromosome has any specific effects on cognitive abilities. It must be remembered that most of these triple-X cases were found in institutions for the mentally retarded and few with average intelligence were included. Further research is required before it is possible to determine the specific effects of an extra X chromosome on intelligence and psychosexual development. Triple-X females with normal intelligence could provide information about the influence, if any, of an extra X chromosome on specific cognitive abilities and on psychiatric characteristics.

Psychiatric Patients

As mentioned previously, there is considerable evidence for the involvement of genetic factors in the etiology of schizophrenia, manic-depressive psychosis, and senile dementia. The evidence for each will be briefly summarized in the following sections.

SCHIZOPHRENIA

It is generally agreed that the tendency to develop schizophrenia is determined by what Kallmann called "inherited predispositional elements."[47] That schizophrenia is determined at least in part by genetic factors, is supported by family, twin, and adoption studies. Family studies show that expectancy rates for schizophrenia are markedly higher in relatives of schizophrenics than in the general population. Moreover, as the degree of consanguinity increases, so does the likelihood of developing the disorder. In a review of the literature, Jarvik and Deckard[51] found an average rate of 15 percent among first-degree relatives of schizophrenics, while the expectancy rate in the general population was about 1 percent.

The results of twin studies also support genetic theories of schizophrenia. Over the past 40 years, 13 studies were conducted in eight countries and the concordance rates for monozygotic (MZ) twins were consistently higher than those for dizygotic (DZ) twins, the average rates being 51.1 percent and 9.1 percent, respectively.[86] To counter the argument that the higher concordance rates for MZ twins might be due to their more similar environment (for example, parents treating MZ twins more alike than DZ twins) several authors have reported concordance rates for MZ twins reared apart. The average concordance rate for MZ twins reared apart for varying lengths of time is 70.8 percent.[51] Although based on small sample sizes, the results suggest that genetic factors are more important in the etiology of schizophrenia than are common environmental factors.

Finally, several studies reported a significantly higher incidence of psychopathology, i.e., schizophrenia, schizoid, and schizophrenic spectrum disorders, among the children of schizophrenic parents than among those of nonschizophrenic parents, even though both groups of children were raised in foster homes.[87-89] Kety and coworkers[90] studied the biological and adoptive families of schizophrenic adoptees and found a significantly higher incidence of schizophrenia and uncertain schizophrenia among the biological relatives.

The combined evidence of these studies supports the conclusion that genetic factors are important in the development of schizophrenia. Therefore, cytogenetic studies were undertaken to investigate the possibility of chromosomal abnormalities in this psychosis.

Raphael and Shaw[91] found no abnormalities of the autosomes among ten schizophrenic patients but they did find one patient with Klinefelter syndrome (47, XXY). As a result, they carried out a sex chromatin survey on 100 female and 100 male schizophrenic patients and found one triple-X female. The authors also compiled data from several sex chromatin surveys and found that the incidence of anomalies among newborn males was 0.26 percent, while among schizophrenic males it was 0.84 percent. The corresponding frequencies among females were 0.09 percent and 0.50 percent, respectively. Because of the small sample of schizophrenics screened, statistical significance was not reached and no conclusions can be drawn at this time from this study. Judd and Brandkamp[92] examined the chromosomes of 40 adult schizophrenics and found no constant chromosomal abnormality. Vartanyan and Gindilis[93] examined 4,091 women hospitalized for various psychoses and found nine of them to have double Barr bodies. Subsequent cytogenetic analysis of these nine individuals revealed that four of them were 47, XXX and the other five mosaics (46, XX/47, XXX) with the majority of the cells (60% − 80%) having a normal karyotype. All nine had been diagnosed as schizophrenic and no sex chromatin anomalies were found among women with other diagnoses, e.g., manic-depressive illness, epilepsy, and senile psychosis. While the results are suggestive of a link between triple-X chromosome abnormality and schizophrenia in women, it cannot be etiologically implicated in the development of schizophrenia since these individuals account for only a small percentage of the total schizophrenic population. Further, the triple-X karyotype is found in normal fertile women free of mental or somatic aberrations. However, it may be that the presence of the triple-X chromosome constitution exacerbates the manifestation of genetic factors underlying schizophrenia.

MANIC-DEPRESSIVE PSYCHOSIS

The genetics of manic-depressive psychosis have not been investigated either as thoroughly or for as long a period of time as those of schizophrenia; however, there is a growing literature. The data from family, twin and adoption studies implicate genetic factors in the tendency to develop manic-depressive illness, both the unipolar and bipolar types.[52,54,94] Bertelsen and colleagues[95] have compiled the data from eight major twin studies as well as their own investigation and found consistently higher concordance rates for MZ twins than for DZ twins, the average rates being 62.0 percent and 18.2 percent, respectively. It has also been found that the biological parents of manic-depressive adoptees exhibit significantly greater rates of affective disorders than do their foster parents.[96] Family studies have also provided evidence for genetic factors in manic-depressive illness. Specifically, these studies[97-101] have shown a preponderance of affected females over males, a finding also supported by two epidemiological studies[102-103] suggesting X-linked dominant transmission. X-linkage was further strengthened by studies[104-107] showing linkage of manic-depressive illness to two known X chromosome markers (Xg[a] antigen and color blindness, both protan and deutan). However, there is controversy regarding sex-linkage since the positions of these two markers, widely separated on the X chromosome, makes linkage to both unlikely. Further, the distinguishing feature of sex-linked inheritance is the absence of father to son transmission and, yet, several reports have been published showing such transmission.[108-111] The possibility that manic-depressive illness also existed on the materal side in these families was examined but could not account for all such transmissions.[107,108,111] One possible explanation may be that manic-depressive illness is genetically heterogeneous with X-linked dominant inheritance in some families and not in others.

Cytogenetic studies are few and have been largely negative. Ebaugh and coworkers[112] reported a trend for a metacentric No. 1 chromosome to be more common in patients with affective disorder than in patients without diagnosed psychiatric illness. Nielsen, Homma and Bertelsen[113] studied chromosome variations in a group of 55 MZ and 52 DZ twin pairs. Several chromosome variations were discovered but they were no more frequent among twins with manic-depressive disorder than among nonaffected twins. No significant differences were found between MZ and DZ twins with regard to incidence of aneuploidy or chromosome aberrations, such as breaks, dicentric chromosomes, deletions, and translocations. Neither were there significant differences in the frequencies of aneuploidy or chromosome aberrations between twins with manic-depressive disorders and those without manic-depressive psychosis. Escobar[114] also found normal chromosome complements in 25 hospitalized patients with the diagnosis of bipolar affective illness. Applying the G banding procedure, as well as analyzing elongated X chromosomes in a subsample of these patients, normal banding patterns and X chromosome structure were found. However, no information was given as to whether or not these patients had a positive family history of bipolar affective illness and this may be one explanation for no X chromosome abnormalities having been found.

SENILE DEMENTIA, ALZHEIMER TYPE

Senile dementia of the Alzheimer type generally occurs after age 70 and involves a progressive, unremitting mental deterioration accompanied by personality changes. Evidence for genetic factors in the etiology of this disorder comes from family and twin studies dating back over 50 years and the data are compatible with both an autosomal dominant and a multifactorial mode of inheritance.[115] Further, there is specificity of genetic factors for senile dementia, Alzheimer type, rather than a generally increased risk for psychoses.

In the most extensive clinical genetic investigation of senile dementia, Larsson and associates[116] identified index cases from hospital records, field investigated relatives, and found that the morbidity risk for senile dementia among first-degree relatives was 4.3 times higher than the risk for the general population but noted no increase in the frequencies of other mental disorders. Further, not a single case of either Pick disease or presenile Alzheimer dementia was reported, suggesting that senile dementia of the Alzheimer type and presenile Alzheimer dementia were distinct entities. However, on the basis of general population rates and the small size of their sample, one would not expect to find any, and other investigators have reported both Alzheimer disease and senile dementia within the same family.

In another study, Akesson[117] surveyed an entire population in a well-defined area of islands off the cost of Sweden and reported a markedly elevated risk for parents and siblings of patients with Alzheimer senile dementia, and this risk increased with age. The rate for parents 60–70 years was 5.6 percent and rose to 23.1 percent for those over 80 years and the corresponding rates for siblings were 7.1 percent and 30.8 percent.

In the only twin study, Kallmann[118] reported concordance rates of 8 percent for dizygotic twins and 42.8 percent for monozygotic twins, with frequencies of 6.5 percent for siblings and 3 percent for parents.

Thus, family and twin studies provide strong evidence for the involvement of hereditary factors in the etiology of senile dementia. Other evidence has been provided by the work of Stam and Op den Velde[119] studying haptoglobin (Hp) polymorphism distribution. They reported an increased Hp1 gene frequency among patients with senile dementia. Cytogenetic studies have also provided evidence for the involvement of genetic factors in senile dementia. Women with senile dementia distinct from arteriosclerotic (multi-infarct) dementia, showed a significant increase in chromosome loss (hypodiploidy) when compared to normal women of comparable age.[120, 121] This relationship has not been duplicated in men but may be due to the small data base for men and further studies are warranted.

The chromosome findings of increased hypodiploidy in females with senile dementia, as compared to those of an equivalent age but free of dementia, has led to a biobehavioral hypothesis relating chromosome changes to impaired mental functioning in the aged. It is postulated that different degrees of hypodiploidy are associated with individual differences in degree of senile mental decline, and by analogy to the gross physical defects and/or mental retardation which are characteristic consequences of chromosome abnormalities in the developing organism; dementia may be one of the consequences of chromosome abnormalities in the aging individual.

Recently, Heston[122,123] has provided further support for the importance of chromosomal abnormalities. In this study an increased frequency of Down syndrome (extra number 21 chromosome) and hematologic malignancy was found in the families of patients with Alzheimer disease including senile dementia.

While these studies provide evidence for the role of genetic factors in senile dementia, the role of exogenous influences in senile dementia is also being investigated with special attention recently directed toward immunologic factors.[115]

SUMMARY AND CONCLUSIONS

There has been rapid progress in the field of human cytogenetics since the report in 1956 of the correct human diploid chromosome number of 46. The finding that patients with Down syndrome have an extra small acrocentric chromosome and a chromosome complement of 47 gave evidence for the first time of an association between a specific chromosomal abnormality, and mental deficiency. Chromosome investigations have also provided leads to the relationship between chromosomal abnormalities and brain dysfunction as well as congenital abnormalities. However, the mechanism by which abnormal chromosome complements produce their deleterious effects still remains to be elucidated.

Evidence from studies of sex chromosome anomalies suggest that these individuals tend to exhibit a higher incidence of psychopathology than does the general population. Yet, since only a minority of individuals with an abnormal sex chromosome constitution develops psychopathology, other factors must play an important role and the abnormal chromosome complement may provide a state of increased vulnerability to these factors. Chromosome surveys of schizophrenics and manic-depressives are few and those that are available have failed to demonstrate any significant or specific chromosome abnormalities. In senile dementia, a generally increased frequency of chromosome loss, especially in the C group chromosomes, has been reported in women when compared to an age-matched group. The significance of this finding, based on relatively few individuals, remains to be elucidated. It should be pointed out, however, that these chromosome studies were carried out primarily on conventionally stained chromosomes and chromosomal abnormalities, although present, may have been below the limits of the then current cytogenetic methodology.

The recent advances in chromosome staining techniques, i.e. banding, offers the ability to detect structural chromosome rearrangements, e.g. reciprocal translocations and inversions heretofore undetectable. The application of these techniques, the continual refinement of the present techniques, as well as the development of new techniques combined with biochemical investigations, promises to provide new insights into biobehavior relationships.

REFERENCES

1. Sutton WS: The chromosomes in heredity. Biol Bull 4:231−251, 1903
2. Morgan TH: Sex limited inheritance in Drosophila. Science 32:120−122, 1910
3. Sturtevant AH: The linear arrangement of six sex-linked factors in Drosophila, as shown by their mode of association. J Explt Zool 14:43−59, 1913
4. Bridges CB: Sex in relation to chromosomes and genes. Am Naturalist 59:127−137, 1925
5. Tjio JH, Levan A: The chromosome number of man. Hereditas 42:1−6, 1956
6. Hansemann D: Ueber pathologische Mitosen. Arch Pathol Anat Physiol 123:356−370, 1891
7. von Winiwarter H: Etude sur la spermatogenèse humaine. Arch Biol (Liege) 27:97−189, 1912
8. Painter TS: The Y chromosome in mammals. Science 53:503−504, 1921
9. Painter TS: Studies in mammalian spermatogenesis. II. The spermatogenesis of man. J Explt Zool 37:291−335, 1923
10. Hamerton JL: Human Cytogenetics, vol. 1. New York, Academic Press, 1971
11. Ford CE, Hamerton JL: The chromosomes of man. Nature 178:1020−1023, 1956
12. Ford CE, Jacobs PA, Lajha LG: Human somatic chromosomes. Nature 181:1565−1568, 1958
13. Lejeune J, Turpin R, Gautier M: Le mongolisme premier exemple d'aberration autosomique humaine. Ann Génét Hum 1:41−49, 1959
14. Jacobs P, Baikie AG, Court-Brown WM, et al: The somatic chromosomes in mongolism. Lancet 1:710, 1959
15. Lejeune J, Gautier M, Turpin R: Etude des chromosomes somatique de neuf enfants mongoliens. Comptes Rendus de l'Academie des Sciences, Paris, 248:1721−1722, 1959
16. Ford CE, Jones KW, Polani PE, et al: A sex-chromosome anomaly in a case of gonadal dysgenesis (Turner's syndrome). Lancet 1:711−713, 1959
17. Ford CE, Jones KW, Miller OJ, et al: The chromosomes in a patient showing both mongolism and the Klinefelter syndrome. Lancet 1:709−710, 1959
18. Ford CE, Polani PE, Briggs JH, et al: A presumptive human XXY/XX mosaic. Nature 183:1030−1032, 1959
19. Jacobs PA, Strong JA: A case of human intersexuality having a possible XXY sex-determining mechanism. Nature 183:302−303, 1959
20. Hungerford DA, Donnelly AJ, Nowell PC, et al: The chromosome constitution of a human phenotypic intersex. Am J Hum Genet 11:215−236, 1959

21. German JL: DNA synthesis in human chromosomes. Trans NY Acad Sci 24:395−407, 1962
22. Caspersson T, Farber S, Foley GE, et al: Chemical differentiation along metaphase chromosomes. Exptl Cell Res 49:219−222, 1968
23. Caspersson T, Zech L, Johansson C: Differential binding of alkylating fluorochromes in human chromosomes. Exptl Cell Res 60:315−319, 1970
24. Caspersson T, Zech L, Johansson C, et al: Identification of human chromosomes by DNA reacting fluorescing agents. Chromosoma 30:215−227, 1970
25. Ellison JR, Barr HJ: Differences in the quinacrine staining of the chromosomes of a pair of sibling species: Drosophila melanogaster and Drosophila simulans. Chromosoma 34:424−435, 1971
26. Weisblum B, de Haseth P: Quinacrine—a chromosome stain specific for deoxyadenylate-deoxythymidylate-rich regions in DNA. Proc Natl Acad Sci USA 69:629−632, 1972
27. Pardue ML, Gall JG: Chromosomal localization of mouse satellite DNA. Science 168:1356−1358, 1970
28. Arrighi FE, Hsu TC: Localization of heterochromatin in human chromosomes. Cytogenetics 10:81−86, 1971
29. Sumner AT, Evans HJ, Buckland RA: New techniques for distinguishing between human chromosomes. Nature, New Biol 232:31−32, 1971
30. Dutrillaux B, Lejeune J: Sur une nouvelle technique d'analyse du caryotype humain. CR Acad Sci Paris 272:2638−2640, 1971
31. Paris Conference (1971): Standardization in Human Cytogenetics Birth Defects: Original Article Series, VIII: 7, National Foundation, New York, 1972
32. Pearson PL, Bobrow M: Definitive evidence for the short arm of the Y chromosome associating with the X chromosome during meiosis in the human male. Nature (London) 226:959−961, 1970
33. Miller OJ, Miller DA, Allerdice, PW, et al: Quinacrine fluorescent karyotypes of human diploid and heteroploid cell lines. Cytogenetics 10:338−346, 1971
34. Steel CM: Non-identity of apparently similar chromosome aberrations in human lymphoblastoid cell lines. Nature (London) 233:555−556, 1971
35. Rowley JD: The role of cytogenetics in hematology. Blood 48:1−7, 1976
36. Manolov G, Manolova Y: Marker band in one chromosome 14 from Burkitt's lymphomas. Nature (London) 237:33−34, 1972
37. Yunis JJ: High resolution of human chromosomes. Science 191:1268−1270, 1976
37a. Yunis JJ: personal communication
38. Barr ML, Bertram EG: A morphological distinction between neurones of the male and female, and the behavior of the nucleolar satellite during accelerated nucleoprotein synthesis. Nature 163:676, 1949
39. Garrod AE: The Croonian lectures on inborn errors of metabolism, I, II, III, IV. Lancet ii: 1−7, 73−79, 142−148, 214−220, 1908
40. Fölling A: Uber Auscheidung von Phenylbrenz-traubensaure in den Harn als Stoffwechselanomalie in Verbindung mit Imbezillität. Zeitschr f Physiol Chem 227:169−176, 1934
41. Penrose LS: Inheritance of phenylpyruvic amentia. Lancet 2:192−194, 1935

42. Jervis GA: The genetics of phenylpyruvic oligophrenia. J Ment Sci 85:719–762, 1939
43. Jervis GA: Phenylpyruvic oligophrenia (phenylkitonuria). Res Publ Ass Nerv Ment Dis 33:259–282, 1954
44. Fölling A, Mohr OL, Ruud L: Oligophrenia Phenylpyrouvica, a recessive syndrome in man. Norske Videnskapo-Akademi Oslo I Mat-Naturv Klasse 13:1–44, 1945
45. Bickel H, Boscott RJ, Gerrard J: Observations on the biochemical error in phenylketonuria and its dietary control. In Waelsck H (ed): Biochemistry of the Developing Nervous System. New York: Academic Press, 1955, pp 417–430
46. Mitoma C, Auld RM, Udenfriend S: On the nature of enzymatic defect in phenylpyruvic oligophrenia. Proc Soc Exptl Biol 94:634, 1957
47. Kallmann FJ: The genetic theory of schizophrenia: An analysis of 691 schizophrenic twin index families. Am J Psychiatry 103:309–322, 1946
48. Shields J: Summary of the genetic evidence. In Rosenthal D, Kety SS (eds): The transmission of schizophrenia. London: Pergamon Press, 1968, pp 95–126
49. Slater E: A review of earlier evidence on genetic factors in schizophrenia. In Rosenthal D, Kety SS (eds): The transmission of schizophrenia. London: Pergamon Press, 1968, pp 15–26
50. Heston LL: The genetics of schizophrenia and schizoid disease. Science 167:249–256, 1970
51. Jarvik LF, Deckard BS: The Odyssean personality: A survival advantage for carriers of genes predisposing to schizophrenia? Neuropsychobiology 3:179–191, 1977
52. Winokur G, Clayton PJ, Reich T: Manic Depressive Illness. St. Louis, Mosby, 1969
53. Mendlewicz J, Rainer JD: Morbidity risk and genetic transmission in manic-depressive illness. Am J Hum Genet 26:692–701, 1975
54. Gershon ES, Bunney WE, Leckman JF, et al: The inheritance of affective disorders: A review of data and of hypotheses. Behav Genet 6:227–261, 1976
55. Crandall BF, Tarjan G: Genetics of mental retardation. In Sperber MA, Jarvik LF (eds): Psychiatry and Genetics: Psychosocial, Ethical and Legal Considerations. New York, Basic Books, 1976, pp 95–116
56. Hamerton JL: Human Cytogenetics II: Clinical Cytogenetics. New York, Academic Press, 1971
57. Maclean N, Mitchell JM, Harnden DG, et al: A survey of sex-chromosome abnormalities among 4,514 mental defectives. Lancet 1:293, 1962
58. Miller OJ: Sex determination: The sex chromosomes and the sex chromatin pattern. Fertil Steril 13:93, 1962
59. Breg WR, Castilla EE, Miller OJ, et al: Sex chromatin and chromosome studies in 1,562 institutionalized mental defectives. J Pediatr 63:738, 1963
60. Levine H: Clinical Cytogenetics. Boston, Little, Brown and Co., 1971
61. Nora JJ, Fraser FC: Medical Genetics: Principles and Practice. Philadelphia: Lea and Febiger, 1974, p 399
62. Jarvik LF: Genetic modes of transmission relevant to psychopathology. In Sperber MA, Jarvik LF (eds): Psychiatry and Genetics. New York, Basic Books, Inc., 1976, pp 3–40

63. Garron DC: Intelligence among persons with Turner's syndrome. Behav Genet 7:105–127, 1977
64. Money J: Cytogenetic and psychosexual incongruities with a note on space-form blindness. Am J Psychiatry 119:820–827, 1963
65. Garron DC: Sex-linked recessive inheritance of spatial and numerical abilities and Turner's syndrome. Psychol Rev 77:147–152, 1970
66. Silbert A, Wolff PH, Lilienthal J: Spatial and temporal processing in patients with Turner's syndrome. Behav Genet 7:11–22, 1977
67. Stafford RE: Sex differences in spatial visualization as evidence of sex-linked inheritance. Percept Motor Skills 13:428, 1961
68. Hartlage IC: Sex-linked inheritance of spatial ability. Percept Motor Skills 31:610, 1970
69. Bock RC, Kolakowski D: Further evidence of sex-linked major-gene influence on human spatial visualizing ability. Am J Hum Genet 25:1, 1973
70. Money J, Mittenthal S: Lack of personality pathology in Turner's syndrome: Relation to cytogenetics, hormones and physique. Behav Genet 1:43, 1970
71. Stoller RJ: Genetics, constitution, and gender disorder. In Sperber MA, Jarvik LF (eds): Psychiatry and Genetics. New York, Basic Books 1976, pp 41–55
72. Sandberg AA, Koepf GF, Ishihara T, et al: An XYY human male. Lancet 2:488, 1961
73. Court-Brown WM: Males with an XYY sex chromosome complement. J Med Genet 5:341, 1968
74. Jacobs PA, Brunton M, Melville MD, et al: Aggressive behavior, mental sub-normality and the XYY male. Nature 208:1351–1352, 1965
75. Jarvik LF, Klodin V, Matsuyama SS: Human aggression and the extra Y chromosome—fact or fantasy? Am J Psychol 28:674, 1973
76. Hook EB: Behavioral implications of the human XYY genotype. Science 179:139, 1973
77. Valentine GH, McClelland MA, Sergovich FR: The growth and development of four XYY infants. Pediatr 48:583–594, 1971
78. Walzer S, Richmond JB, Gerald PS: The implications of sharing genetic information. In Sperber MA, Jarvik LF (eds): Psychiatry and Genetics. New York, Basic Books, 1976, pp 147–162
79. Haka-Ikse K, Stewart DA, Cripps MH: Early development of children with sex chromosome aberrations. Pediatr 62:761–766, 1978
80. Owen DR: The XYY male: A review. Psychol Bull 78:209, 1972
81. Tzoneva-Maneva MT, Bosajieva E, Petrov B: Chromosomal abnormalities in idiopathic osteoarthropathy. Lancet 1:1000–1002, 1966
82. Sundequist U, Hellstrom E: Transmission of 47, XYY karyotype? Lancet 2:1367, 1969
83. Thompson H, Melnyk J, Hecht F: Reproduction and meiosis in XYY. Lancet 2:831, 1967
84. Diario RB, Glass RH: The Y chromosome in sperm of an XYY male. Lancet 2:1318–1319, 1970
85. Chandley AC, Fletcher J, Robinson JA: Normal meiosis in two 47, XYY men. Hum Genet 33:231–240, 1976
86. Liston EH, Jarvik LF: Genetics of schizophrenia. In Sperber MA, Jarvik LF

(eds): Psychiatry and Genetics. New York, Basic Books, 1976, pp 76—94

87. Heston LL: Psychiatric disorders in foster home reared children of schizophrenic mothers. Br J Psychiatry 112:819—825, 1966

88. Rosenthal D, Wender PH, Kety SS, et al: The adopted-away offspring of schizophrenics. Am J Psychiatry 128:307—311, 1971

89. Kety SS, Rosenthal D, Wender PH, et al: Mental illness in biological and adoptive families of adopted individuals who have become schizophrenic: A preliminary report based upon psychiatric interviews. In Fieve R, Rosenthal D, Brill H (eds): Genetic Research in Psychiatry. Baltimore, John Hopkins University Press, 1975, pp 147—165

90. Kety SS, Rosenthal D, Wender PH, et al: Mental illness in the biological and adoptive families of adopted individuals who have become schizophrenic. Behav Genet 6:219—225, 1976

91. Raphael T, Shaw MW: Chromosome studies in schizophrenia. J Am Med Assoc 183:1022—1028, 1963

93. Judd LL, Brandkamp WW: Chromosome analyses of adult schizophrenics. Arch Gen Psychiatry 16:316—324, 1967

93. Vartanyan ME, Gindilis VM: The role of chromosomal aberrations in the clinical polymorphism of schizophrenia. Int J Ment Health 1:93—106, 1972

94. Cadoret RJ, Winokur, G: Genetics of affective disorders. In Sperber MA, Jarvik LF (eds): Psychiatry and Genetics. New York, Basic Books, 1976, pp 66—75

95. Bertelsen A, Harvald B, Hauge M: A Danish twin study of manic-depressive disorders. Br J Psychiatry 130:330—351, 1977

96. Mendlewicz J, Rainer JD: Adoption study supporting genetic transmission in manic-depressive illness. Nature 268:327—329, 1977

97. Winokur G, Pitts FN Jr: Affective disorder, VI. A family history study of prevalence, sex differences and possible genetic factors. J Psychiat Res 3:113—123, 1965

98. Gershon ES, Mark A, Cohen N, et al: Transmitted factors in the morbid risk of affective disorders: A controlled study. J Psychiat Res 12:283—300, 1975

99. Goetz U, Green R, Whybrow P, et al: X-linkage revisited—A further family history study of manic-depressive illness. Arch Gen Psychiatry 31:665—672, 1974

100. Stendstedt A: A study of manic-depressive psychosis. Acta Psychiat Neurol Scand 79 (Suppl):111, 1952

101. Perris C: A study of bipolar (manic depressive) and unipolar recurrent depressive psychoses. Acta Psychiat Scand 194 (Suppl):420, 1966

102. Helgason T: Epidemiology of mental disorders in Iceland. Acta Psychiat Scand 40 (Suppl 173):1—258, 1964

103. Fremming KH: The Expedtation of Mental Infirmity in a Sample of the Danish Population. London, Cassell, 1951

104. Reich T, Clayton PJ, Winokur G: Family history studies, V. The genetics of mania. Am J Psychiatry 125:1358—1370, 1969

105. Winokur G, Tanna VL: Possible role of X-linked dominant factor in manic-depressive disease. Dis Nerv Syst 30:89—93, 1969

106. Mendlewicz J, Fleiss JL, Fieve RR: Evidence for X-linkage in the transmission of manic-depressive illness. J Am Med Assoc 222:1624–1627, 1972
107. Fieve RR, Mendlewicz J, Fleiss JJ: Manic-depressive illness: Linkage with the Xg^a blood group. Am J Psychiatry 130:1355–1359, 1973
108. Von Grieff H, McHugh PR, Stokes P: The familial history in sixteen males with bipolar manic-depressive disorder. Paper presented at 63rd annual meeting, American Psychopathological Association, New York, 1973
109. Perris C: Genetic transmission of depressive psychoses. Acta Psychiatr Scand 203 (Suppl):45–52, 1968
110. Dunner D, Gershon E, Goodwin FK: Heritable factors in the severity of affective illness. Paper presented at 123rd annual meeting of the American Psychiatric Association, San Francisco, 1970
111. Green R, Goetze V, Whybrow P, et al: X-linked transmission of manic-depressive illness. J Am Med Assoc 223:1289, 1973
112. Ebaugh IA Jr, Freiman M, Woolf RB, et al: Chromosome studies in patients with affective disorder (manic-depressive illness). Arch Gen Psychiatr 19:751–752, 1968
113. Nielsen J, Homma A, Bertelsen A: Cytogenetic investigation in twins with manic-depressive disorders (22 monozygotic and 27 dizygotic twin pairs). Br J Psychiatry 130:352–354, 1977
114. Escobar JI: A cytogenetic study of bipolar affective illness. Comprehen Psychiatry 19:331–335, 1978
115. Matsuyama SS, Jarvik LF: Genetics and mental functioning in senescence. In Birren JE, Sloane B (eds): Handbook of Mental Health and Aging. New Jersey Prentice-Hall, 1980, pp 134–148
116. Larsson T, Sjogren T, Jacobson G: Senile dementia: A clinical sociomedical and genetic study. Acta Psychiatr Scand 39 (Suppl):1–259, 1963
117. Akesson HO: A population study of senile and arteriosclerotic psychoses. Hum Hered 19:546–566, 1969
118. Kallmann FJ: Heredity in Health and Mental Disorder. New York, W.W. Norton, 1953
119. Stam FC, Op den Velde W: Haptoglobin types in Alzheimer's disease and senile dementia. In Katzman R, Terry RD, Bick KL (eds): Alzheimer's Disease: Senile Dementia and Related Disorders (Aging, vol. 7). New York, Raven Press, 1978, pp 279–286
120. Nielsen J: Chromosomes in senile, presenile, and arteriosclerotic dementia. J Gerontol 25:312–315, 1970
121. Jarvik LF, Altshuler KZ, Kato T, et al: Organic brain syndrome and chromosome loss in aged twins. Dis Nerv Syst 32:159–170, 1971
122. Heston LL: Alzheimer's disease, trisomy 21, and myeloproliferative disorders: Associations suggesting a genetic diathesis. Science 196:322–323, 1976
123. Heston LL, Mastri AR: The genetics of Alzheimer's disease: Associations with hematologic malignancy and Down's syndrome. Arch Gen Psychiatry 34:976–981, 1977

Marvin Karno

2
Schizophrenia

The generic title "research in practice" suggests a unidirectional flow of influence, that is, that the published findings of scientific research do influence or should influence the direct treatment of patients. The practice of psychiatry in the past 100 years, however, has been compelled, in the face of the enormous scope of human suffering, disability and tragedy induced by schizophrenic disorders, to try to do something to help. In this regard, the psychiatric profession has had to face the same historical demands as the rest of the medical profession—to act without or with only the most primitive scientific guidelines. It would seem reasonable that the current and continuing findings of an explosively developing international scientific research inquiry into the nature of schizophrenia should be lending support to at least some of the established principles of treatment practice that are regarded by skilled and experienced clinicians as essential, and that derived from long years of pragmatic trial and error. Thus, a two-way traffic of influence should be demonstrable between research findings and treatment practice.

A third source of experience should provide a degree of independent validation for certain findings of both investigators and clinicians, this third source being the personal experience of those who have suffered from schizophrenic illness and who have had the skill and motivation to meaningfully identify and communicate both about the nature of their experience and about what has helped or hindered their episodes of remission and periods of sustained recovery.

It is then the intent of this discussion, which is presented from the perspective of a psychiatric clinician and generalist, to identify a few selected aspects of schizophrenic disorder for which a triangulated continuity of potential understanding and confirmation can be identified between illness-experience, treatment-principles and biobehavioral research findings. Although the emphasis will be on implications for treatment, this discussion will begin with some research findings.

RESEARCH FINDINGS

At the second International Conference on Schizophrenia, hosted by Rochester University in May of 1976, in conjunction with the Conference on Attention and Information Processing sponsored by the Scottish Rite Schizophrenic Research Program, the state of the art in research on schizophrenia at that time was publicly presented. It appeared in print in 1978 in the form of 61 papers published by John Wiley as The Nature of Schizophrenia: New Approaches to Research and Treatment.[1] Fully 25 of the 61 papers focus on psychophysiologic measurements of perception, attention, arousal, visual tracking, and reaction time in schizophrenic patients.

Such measurements, for example reaction time, date back as far as 1868 in the study of psychological processes.[2] In regard to more recent research into the nature of schizophrenia, the focus upon disordered perception, sensation, and attention presupposes a conceptual model of a fundamental neurophysiological disturbance in what has recently come to be generically called *information processing*.

As summarized by Spring and Zubin,[3] "Disturbances of information processing have a prima-facie link with the schizophrenic psychopathologic state because patients' subjective complaints so often include altered perceptual experience, distractibility, and flooding or loss of the ability to differentiate figure from ground. Even if these disturbances do not produce or cause schizophrenia, they may serve as 'culture-free' markers of that disorder or of vulnerability to it."

I will briefly review a few of these components of information processing which have been repeatedly and consistently found to be defective or disordered in persons subject to schizophrenia. The method of reaction time (RT) was developed by Shakow and colleagues over 40 years ago and consists of measuring the time lapse between stimulus and response of subjects under differing experimental conditions. During and between episodes of active psychosis, persons suffering from schizophrenia have been found to be slow in reaction time, and most importantly, they are not benefited by being given a regular, predictable preparatory interval between a warning stimulus and an imperative stimulus in the testing situation. Schizophrenics are also characteristically impaired to a disproportionate degree when reaction time is tested with shorter, irregular preparatory intervals. Later work by Rodnick and Shakow[4] led to the development of a "set index" which subsumed specific RT deficits found in schizophrenics and which discriminated chronic schizophrenics from non-schizophrenics. Cancro has regarded the RT studies as ". . . the closest thing to a north star in schizophrenia research."[5]

Deficits or abnormalities in attention have long been studied among persons suffering from schizophrenia. Bleuler observed that "the facilitating as well as the inhibiting properties of attention are equally disturbed" in schizophrenia.[6] He noted that active attention might be severely restricted in withdrawn patients except for an area of focus, e.g., "An apathetic schizophrenic can concentrate for half a day all his small strength on a little thread which he holds in his hand. On the other hand, he may be diverted by every trifle, because no interest to speak of restrains him."[7]

Bleuler was dramatically impressed by the powers of passive and apparently nonselective registration of information among their schizophrenic patients. "Events on the ward which did in no way refer to the patients, newspaper reports which they heard only in passing, can be reproduced after years in every detail by patients who appeared completely absorbed in themselves who always sat gazing into some corner, so that one can hardly understand how these people managed to learn of these matters."[8]

Distractibility has been repeatedly measured as one parameter of a presumed attentional deficit in schizophrenia. This has usually involved the comparison of performances by schizophrenic and control subjects in what are called neutral and distractor conditions. For example, in a neutral test condition, subjects would hear a tape-recorded female voice reading a list of simple digits and would then be asked to write down the digits from memory after the recording. In the distractor condition, irrelevant digits would be read by a recorded male voice in the intervals between the relevant digits read by the female voice. Subjects would be told to ignore the male voice and only remember and write down the digits read by the female voice. Schizophrenics do significantly poorer than nonschizophrenics in the distractor but not in the neutral condition. This suggests a specific defect in the capacity to screen or filter out distracting stimuli in schizophrenia. Of particular interest is that recent, carefully designed work has shown that antipsychotic medication produces near normal distraction responses among schizophrenics but that off medication, persons suffering from schizophrenia show a dramatic deterioration, i.e., greatly heightened distractibility, but are still equal to normals in the nondistracted, neutral recall task.[9] Most interestingly according to one recent study, if only research diagnostic criteria (RDC) -positive schizophrenic patients, excluding those diagnosed as schizoaffective, are compared to nonschizophrenic controls, then even antipsychotic medication does not restore the test scores of the schizophrenic patients to normal. The Research

Diagnostic Criteria[10] were devised by Spitzer and his colleagues to include explicit inclusion and exclusion criteria for arriving at specific psychiatric diagnoses; the criteria for schizo-affective disorder incorporate the common overlapping patterns of combined affective and thought disorder symptoms. Thus rigorously (RDC) diagnosed schizophrenic patients show heightened distractibility even when maintained on antipsychotic medication.[11]

Two other tests used to measure the ability to maintain attention over time are the Continuous Performance Test and the Span of Apprehension Task. The Continuous Performance Test involves the presentation of randomly arranged numbers or letters on a screen at a rate of about one every second. They are shown for a fraction of a second, and the subject is instructed to press a button immediately after certain preselected target stimuli are presented. The number and kinds of errors as well as correct responses are scored. The Span of Apprehension Task requires subjects to observe a screen on which zero to nine letters are very briefly projected. The subjects are instructed to note and report verbally which of two preselected target letters are projected along with the nontarget letters. The number of nontarget or competing and irrelevant stimuli are gradually increased, so that the information processing and selecting demands of the test are gradually increased. Again, errors and correct responses are scored.

Both of these tests (CPT & SPAN) have consistently demonstrated deficits in schizophrenics compared to nonschizophrenics, although a recent report has indicated that antipsychotic medication tends to normalize the scores of schizophrenics on both these tests as well as on reaction time, and that clinical improvement correlates with improvement in information processing.[12]

I will only very briefly mention Holzman's interesting findings that smooth pursuit eye movements show defective or abnormal patterns in schizophrenics. These patterns are not unique to schizophrenics, but one form, called Type II by Holzman, has so far been found in patients with multiple sclerosis, Parkinson's disease, brain-stem and hemispheric lesions, in states of drug intoxication, and in schizophrenics. The abnormality is found in schizophrenics not on medication, and in about 45 percent of nonclinically ill first-degree relatives of schizophrenics. Disordered smooth pursuit eye movements have been found in only 6 percent of normal subjects, but 65 percent to 80 percent of schizophrenic patients.[13]

Smooth pursuit refers to the movement of the eyes in following a moving object such as a pendulum, in order to maintain the moving image on the fovea. Saccadic movements keep bringing the image back onto the fovea.

Of importance for the present discussion is that smooth pursuit appears to be an essentially nonvoluntary component of attentional behavior and therefore may be a component of what is, broadly speaking, information-processing. In this case, the registration of information. Holzman has presented arguments for the belief that this defect represents an impaired neurophysiologic substrate within the central nervous system.[13]

In summary, from the few examples cited and from a huge research literature which has not been cited, it appears that persons suffering from schizophrenia show difficulty in sorting out relevant from irrelevant stimuli, respond more slowly to relevant stimuli, show a decrease rather than an increase in performance under conditions of high arousal, and in general show a lower than normal threshold for overload in situations of information processing.

SUBJECTIVE EXPERIENCES

I would now like to shift the reader's attention to a consideration of some of the subjective experiences of schizophrenic illness which appear congruent with the psychopathological findings which have been described. For any who have not read it, Barbara J. Freedman's March 1974 report in the Archives of General Psychiatry[14] is a superb anthology of autobiographical accounts. For richness of detail, James Chapman's 1966 abstract of his M.D. thesis (in the British Journal of Psychiatry) on the Early Symptoms of Schizophrenia,[15] should be read and reread by every psychiatrist.

Regarding the well known symptom of Blocking, Chapman carefully interviewed his subjects, and recorded verbatim accounts. A 31-year-old, single male bricklayer reported "It's like a temporary blackout—with my brain not working properly . . . I just get cut off from outside things and go into another world. This happens when the tension starts to mount until it bursts in my brain. It has to do with what is going on around me—taking in too much of my surroundings . . . I can't shut things out of my mind and everything closes in on me. It stops me thinking and then the mind goes a blank and everything gets switched off. I can't retain anything for any length of time—only a few seconds, and I can't do simple habits like walking or cleaning my teeth. I have to use all my mind to do these things . . . I can't control what's coming in and it stops me thinking with the mind a blank."

A 24-year-old single male apprentice accountant reported "I don't like dividing my attention at any time because it lends to confusion and I don't know where I am or who I am. When this starts . . . I just turn off all my senses and I don't see anything and I don't hear anything . . . It's all right if it's just one thing at a time but I am virtually blind at these times and can't move properly because there are so many things coming into my eyes that I don't know what's what . . . I can't work myself."

A 21-year-old single, apprentice slater reports: "Nothing settles in my mind—not even for a second . . . My mind goes away—too many things come into my head at once and I lose control . . . I'm falling apart into bits. My mind is not right if I walk and speak. It's better to stay still and not say a word.''[15]

These accounts of subjective information flooding, leading to blanking out or the sensation of fragmentation of the self by Chapman's subjects, are compatible with Norma MacDonald's account of ''Living with Schizophrenia,'' which first appeared in a 1960 issue of the Canadian Medical Association Journal. In writing of her illness, she describes ''At first it was as if parts of my brain 'awoke' which had been dormant, and I became interested in a wide assortment of people, events, places and ideas which normally would make no impression on me . . . Every face in the windows of a passing streetcar would be engraved in my mind . . . Now, many years later, I can appreciate what had happened. Each of us is capable of coping with a large number of stimuli, invading our being through any one of the senses. We could hear every sound within earshot and see every object, line, and color within the field of vision, and so on. It's obvious that we would be incapable of carrying on any of our daily activities if even one-hundredth of all these available stimuli invaded us at once. So the mind must have a filter which functions without our conscious thought, sorting stimuli and allowing only those which are relevant to the situation in hand to disturb consciousness. And this filter must be working at maximum efficiency at all times, particularly when we require a high degree of concentration. What had happened to me . . . was a breakdown in the filter, and a hodge-podge of unrelated stimuli were distracting me from things which should have had my undivided attention . . . My brain . . . had become sore with a real physical soreness, as if it had been rubbed with sandpaper until it was raw . . . I had very little ability to sort the relevant from the irrelevant . . . the filter had broken down.''[16]

Freedman notes from her review of over 50 autobiographical books and articles by persons afflicted with schizophrenia that ''Problems in focusing attention and concentrating were mentioned more often than any other cognitive or perceptual disorder by these patients.'' Freedman cites a report by Coate, writing about schizophrenics like herself, ''it is not that he cannot keep to the point, but that there are so many points, and all equally and insistently insignificant, like a starlit sky with 50 different pole stars in the sky.''[14]

It would be boringly redundant but remarkable for the detailed similarity involved, to recount other narrative descriptions of what we may refer to as information processing overload in persons suffering from schizophrenia; similar subjective confirmation exists for distractibility, dramatic variations in sensory perception, speeding up or slowing of thoughts, a sense of loss of meaning of familiar words, objects and persons, and a host of other distortions of the normally ordered flow and patterning of subjective mental experience in schizophrenia. All experienced clinicians have had their patients share these painful experiences with them on many occasions.

PSYCHOTHERAPEUTIC TREATMENT

Certain accounts of what has been found helpful in the psychotherapeutic treatment of schizophrenia are relevant to the foregoing presentation.

In the April, 1946 issue of the Psychiatric Quarterly, John N. Rosen's first paper appeared, reporting a psychotherapeutic method of rapidly and effectively treating three young patients in states of acute catatonic excitement, which he had carried out on an intuitive basis while a resident at the Brooklyn State Hospital in 1943. Rosen's technique, which he called "direct psychoanalysis" achieved considerable acclaim, fame and skepticism during the final decade before the advent of effective antipsychotic pharmacologic agents and this author suggests that there are specific aspects to his work which indicate that he was effective for reasons probably unrelated to the degree of validity of his own theoretical formulations.

Rosen described direct analysis as "a psychologic technique having for its purpose the treatment and care of psychotic patients."[17a] He regarded as the essential principle ". . . that the therapist must be a loving, omnipotent protector and provider for the patient."[17b] The specific psychotherapeutic maneuvers which he used initially on an intuitive basis and which he only later became consciously aware of, included direct interpretations, direct transference interpretations, confronting and overcoming the patients' aggressions, the use of safe, pleasant settings, and direct participation in the patients' psychotic experience.

Regarding direct interpretation, Rosen writes: "When the patient is mute, he is generally rigid. In that case, it must be understood that what the patient is saying is 'I am frightened stiff.' You have to tell him just so that you understand this. It is necessary for the therapist to utilize that aspect of the hallucination, delusion, gesticulation, or whatever, to select that remark or act which, in the light of what we know about psychosis in general and this patient's psychosis in particular seems most obvious as expressing in this peculiar way some direct need of the patient. You must tell him what you see or hear him to be saying so that somewhere, inside of him, he will gain the sense that he is no longer alone; he is understood. Somebody . . . is trying to help. Somebody will give him what he cannot get by himself."[17c] In regard to a male patient who was using his engineering background to discover a more powerful fluid automotive transmission than any yet invented, Rosen told the patient that he was trying to determine "How can you transmit mother's milk to your mouth?'' The patient responded, ''My mother thought I always needed a vacation.'' Rosen's reply, ''Anything to get rid of you.''[17d]

Rosen engaged in remarkably dramatic, intense relationships with schizophrenic patients. He believed that schizophrenia was induced by toxic parenting and that it was the final stage in a retreat from reality, which went through a sequence of general neurotic, obsessive-compulsive, manic-depressive, and paranoid layers before the final stage of schizophrenia. He believed that the psychic conflictual experiences in early life which led to the regression to schizophrenia could be undone psychologically and that direct psychoanalysis represented a psycho-therapeutic reparenting which could then produce a normal individual.

Although Rosen's theoretical positions might find few sources of support today, his techniques deserve reexamination. I believe that he demonstrated a rare gift of being able to powerfully engage and sustain the attention of schizophrenic patients, to communicate with them in strong, simple language indicating comprehension of their inner states of confusion and terror as well as a comprehension and acceptance of their delusional and hallucinatory experiences. I do not think it far-fetched to suppose that Rosen's involvement tended to prioritize competing perceptual stimulation, unload informational overload, provide adequate time for appropriate reaction, and shut out irrelevant competing stimulation, while conveying an awesome sense of rescue and hope.

Although a five year follow-up study of the results of direct analysis compared to other forms of treatment of first-episode schizophrenic patients was reported as showing no advantage to Rosen's controversial methods,[18] a later review of that study pointed out the many methodological deficiencies which rendered its findings inconclusive. The short-term dramatic effectiveness of Rosen's work has been witnessed and documented by respected clinicians, and Feinsilver and Gunderson have appropriately cited Fromm-Reichmann's observation that the essential benefit of the direct method is not cure of schizophrenia but rather the rapid resolution of episodes of acute psychosis.[19]

Rosen commented about his work, ''Once the initial investment of interest, effort and time is made, the agreeable or disagreeable qualities of the patient are not the factors that sustain the therapist in his devotion. The patient has become like a member of your family and you have to respond to the needs of the patient on that basis. But there are other aspects in your relationships to members of your family. In no healthy family is love the only feeling. You begin to fight with the patient; you withdraw from the patient, you no longer make the same sacrifice for him. The therapist does many things to diminish the intensity of the feeling after the needs of the patient have diminished.''[17e]

In 1954 Barbara Betz and John C. Whitehorn published their studies on the relationship between characteristics of physician psychotherapists and the clinical outcome of their schizophrenic patients.[20] They reviewed the records of 14 resident psychiatrists in their treatment of a combined total of 100 schizophrenic patients at the Johns Hopkins' Phipps Clinic in the pre-phenothiazine years, 1944 to 1952. This sample was obtained by screening 35 residents, whose improvement rates for their treated schizophrenic patients as measured by daily nursing observations, averaged 50.6 percent, with a range of zero to 100 percent.

The seven highest-ranking residents (with a range of 68 to 100 percent, averaging 75 percent improvement) were selected as Group A. Group B consisted of the seven residents with the lowest improvement ratings, that is, a range of zero to 34 percent, averaging 27 percent. (Their combined 103 schizophrenic patients were rounded off to 100 by omitting the 3 with shortest hospital stay records). Of the 100 patients, 48 were treated by Group A physicians and 52 by Group B physicians.

Improvement was evaluated by review of disposition at discharge, social participation, participation in activity programs, and behavioral chartings. The findings were as follows:[20]

1. Patients who improved did not differ in severity of illness from patients who did not improve.
2. Group A therapists did not differ from Group B therapists in results with nonschizophrenic patients, i.e., they were not better therapists in general.
3. Patients tended to improve when their physicians indicated some grasp of the personal meaning and motivation of the patients' behavior.
4. Patients tended to improve when their physicians selected personality-rather than psychopathology-oriented goals, i.e., when the physician aimed at assisting the patient in definite modifications of personal adjust-ment patterns and toward more constructive use of assets rather than mere decrease of symptoms or vague "better socialization".
5. Patients tended to improve when their physicians in day-to-day encounters used active personal participation rather than passive-permissive or in-terpretive approaches.
6. Patient's improvement was highly associated with their development of trusting, confidential relationships with their physician therapists.

It seems reasonable to conclude that Whitehorn and Betz support the importance of direct, personal engagement with explicit communication, posi-tive regard, and avoidance of the potential informational overload of a psychodynamic-interpretive nature. The Group A physicians identified by Betz and Whitehorn intuitively tended to supply an exogenous filter in their communications with their patients. Rosen's therapeutic work, operating from a somewhat uniquely authoritarian and intensive basis, did much the same.

Turning to the work of Richard Lamb in the long-term psychotherapeutic management of schizophrenia in association with active pharmacologic treatment, we find a master of the art of clarity, conciseness, directness, engagement and caring. Like most who work with schizophrenia, he not infrequently gives direct advice.

The insight which Lamb advocates for the schizophrenic is into the connections between sources of stress, usually interpersonal, and the symptoms experienced. The patient is taught to recognize the predictable occurrence of symptom exacerbation in certain life situations, and what change the patient can make in his interactions with family and friends to decrease the frequency and intensity of such experiences.

The clinical account of his, which is my favorite, is the following:[21]

"A 36-year old married woman had been hospitalized five times for acute psychotic episodes . . . but for five years she had been doing well in outpatient psychotherapy. She was on vacation, visiting her mother in another city, when she called her therapist, obviously disturbed and in the incipient stage of a psychotic episode. . . . the therapist ascertained that she had been going through her mother's cedar chest [and] . . . had come across a birthday card she had received from her late father on her 11th birthday, on which he had written, 'Happy birthday to a good little girl who is doing the dishes on her own birthday.' She was flooded with memories of the deprivation she had experienced as a child, of the unreasonable demands that had been placed on her, and of the feelings of loss for her dead father, about whom she felt ambivalent. The therapist's response was, 'Put all those things back and close that cedar chest.' The patient complied, and when she called back an hour later she was much less distraught; she now felt in control of the situation, and a psychotic decompensation had been averted. In succeeding visits over the years she did not reopen the cedar chest, either literally or figuratively." Lamb summarizes that "Nothing is more difficult for many therapists than to give direct advice . . . in simple language without jargon."

Those who have been working over time with schizophrenic patients will, no doubt, have had similar experiences. I have worked with a small number of chronic schizophrenic patients (for, on the average, seven years each), and they have convinced me of their distractibility, their sensitive vulnerability to situations of high stimulation or strongly competing demands, their defective capacity to filter out irrelevant input in contexts of stress, and their morale-shattering tendency to experience a rapid escalation of psychotic symptoms when under excessive stress. We learn that these patients are able to compensate rapidly and dramatically after resumed or increased medication, practical advice concerning situations of stress, the conveying of concern, positive regard and hope, and the ready availability of further contact if and when needed. These are modes of response which unload overload; they engage and focus attention, encourage thinking and problem-solving, and replace terror and despair with relief and hope.

The characteristic deficits of psychobiological functioning which have been found to characterize schizophrenia have been documented by the earliest astute clinicians, by patients themselves, and by laboratory investigations utilizing careful, scientific design. The understanding of the nature and extent of these handicaps is still extremely limited, but through future concerted effort from these three sources of experience, this understanding can expand to allow us to better help the schizophrenic patient.

REFERENCES

1. Wynne, LC, Cromwell, RL, Matthysse S. (eds): The Nature of Schizophrenia: New Approaches to Research and Treatment. New York, Wiley, 1978
2. Spring B, Zubin J: Reaction time and attention in schizophrenia: A comment on K.H. Nuechterlein's critical evaluation of the data and theories. Schizophrenia Bulletin 3:437−444, 1977
3. Spring B, Zubin J: Attention and information processing as indicators of vulnerability to schizophrenic episodes, in Wynne LC, Cromwell RL, Matthysse S. (eds): The Nature of Schizophrenia: New Approaches to Research and Treatment. New York, Wiley, 1978, p 366
4. Rodnick E, Shakow D: Set in the schizophrenic as measured by a composite reaction time index. Am J Psychiat 97:214−225, 1940
5. Cancro R, Sutton S, Keer J, et al: Reaction time and prognosis in acute schizophrenia. J Nerv Ment Dis 153:352, 1971
6. Bleuler E: Dementia Praecox or the Group of Schizophrenias. New York, International Universities Press, 1950, p 68
7. Bleuler E: Textbook of Psychiatry. New York, Macmillan, 1924, p 134
8. Bleuler E: Dementia Praecox or the Group of Schizophrenias. New York, International Universities Press, 1950, p 68−69
9. Spohn HE, Lacoursiere RB, Thompson K, et al: Phenothiazine effects on psychological and psychophysiological dysfunction in chronic schizophrenics. Arc Gen Psychiat 34:633−644, 1977
10. Spitzer RL, Endicott J, Robins E: Research Diagnostic Criteria (RDC) for a Selected Group of Functional Disorders. New York, Biometrics Research, 1975, pp 6−12
11. Oltmanns TF, Ohayon J, Neale JM: The effect of antipsychotic medication and diagnostic criteria on distractibility in schizophrenia, in Wynne LC, Cromwell RL, Matthysse S. (eds.): The Nature of Schizophrenia: New Approaches to Research and Treatment. New York, Wiley, 1978, p 283
12. Spohn HE, Lacoursiere RB, Thompson K, et al: The effects of antipsychotic drug treatment on attention and information processing in chronic schizophre-

nics, in Wynne LC, Cromwell RL, Matthysse S. (eds): The Nature of Schizo-phrenia: New Approaches to Research and Treatment. New York, Wiley, 1978, p 280

13. Holzman PS, Levy DL, Proctor LR: The several qualities of attention in schizo-phrenia, in Wynne LC, Cromwell RL, Matthysse S. (eds): The Nature of Schiz-ophrenia: New Approaches to Research and Treatment. New York, Wiley, 1978, pp 295–306

14. Freedman BJ: The subjective experience of perceptual and cognitive distur-bances in schizophrenia: A review of autobiographical accounts. Arch Gen Psychiat 30:333–340, 1974

15. Chapman J: The early symptoms of schizophrenia. Brit J Psychiat 112:225–251, 1966

16. MacDonald N: Living with schizophrenia. Can Med Assoc J 82:218–221, 678–681, 1960

17. Rosen JN: Direct Analysis: General principles in Rosen JN: Direct Analysis: Selected papers. New York, Grune and Stratton, 1953, (a) p 1; (b) p 8; (c) p 13; (d) p 14; (e) p 11

18. Brookhammer RS, Meyers RW, Schober CC,: A five year follow-up study of schizophrenics treated by Rosen's "direct analysis": Compared with controls. Amer J Psychiat 123:602–604, 1966

19. Feinsilver DB, Gunderson JG: Psychotherapy for schizophrenics—is it indi-cated? A review of the relevant literature. Schizophrenia Bulletin 6:11–23, 1972

20. Whitehorn JC, Betz BJ: A study of psychotherapeutic relationships between physicians and schizophrenic patients. Amer J Psychiat 111:321–331, 1954

21. Lamb R: Helping the long-term schizophrenic. Psychiat Annals 5:279–285, 1975

E. A. Serafetinides

3

Psychopathology and the Cerebral Hemispheres

This author's first involvement with studies on cerebral lateralization was in 1964, when he and his associates reported on the significance of hemispheric laterality for the maintenance of consciousness in human subjects.[1-3] Findings on the significance of cerebral dominance in other psychological phenomena, such as aggressiveness, psychedelic effects, memory and emotions, followed.[4-9] Lastly, findings on the symmetry of EEG phenomena in psychosis were reported in the 1970s.[10-15] Lateralization of cerebral functions is, of course, nothing new in medicine; a considerable portion of neurology is based on such observations. What is new is the attention cerebral lateralization is getting in psychiatry and the behavioral sciences. In the last few years alone, the literature on hemispheric functions has grown enormously. The purpose of this chapter, then, is not to attempt a cursory review of this subject (the reader should refer to a number of books and monographs published recently, e.g. references [16-24]), but to selectively discuss pertinent characteristics of the electrophysiology (EEG and evoked responses) of hemispheric functions as they may apply to psychiatric conditions.

PSYCHOPATHOLOGY AND BRAIN ELECTROPHYSIOLOGY

In general, the literature on brain electrophysiology and psychopathology is characterized by certain notions on which most investigators appear to agree. These are, in brief: there is no gross or exclusive signature (i.e. in the manner of seizure EEG discharges) that can be detected by the unaided eye and can be considered pathognomonic of any specific psychopathological condition; nonspecific abnormalities can be seen in various conditions but by themselves they are of little diagnostic or prognostic significance. A number of claims have been advanced regarding the presence of either scalp recorded specific patterns (e.g. B-mitten or positive spikes, etc.) or depth recorded specific findings (e.g. septal spikes) in certain conditions, the significance of which is still a matter of discussion if not controversy. Finally, a number of new techniques (e.g. AER, computer and activation techniques of EEG analysis, etc.) are increasingly being used as promising new tools in this area, suggesting the existence of quantifiable and/or lateralized findings in relation to psychopathology.[10-15,25,26]

We shall review here those reports in the literature which not only deal with interhemispheric observations but also do it in a quantified way. The first reports in this context showed evidence of greater interhemispheric symmetry in active schizophrenics.[10,11,27] In 1973, for example, Sugarman, et al reported decreased right sided amplitude in instances of dreaming and in some psychiatric conditions, and interpreted this to mean as signifying involvement of the right or nondominant hemisphere in these instances (reduced amplitude, signifying, in its turn, activation of said hemisphere).[28]

Analyses of the EEG amplitude levels (integrative method) in the right (R) and left (L) occipital areas of human subjects reveal that there exists in most subjects a R/L difference; however, Goldstein and Stolzfus showed that in terms of existing R/L EEG amplitude differences certain psychoactive drugs can change the normal lateralization patterns.[29] Thus, stimulants tend to decrease interhemispheric differences, while following drug-induced euphoria these differences are increased. Also, hallucinogens can reverse lateralization while neuroleptics produce a decrease in the variability of amplitude ratios. No changes are seen with sedatives, minor tranquilizers and placebo. Another way of interpreting these changes is to consider that non-specific arousal or activation creates symmetry through bilateral reduction of amplitude and emergence of fast rhythms, whereas selective activation, as with hallucinogenic drugs, or relaxation, where natural dominance patterns operate unhindered, allow the interhemispheric asymmetries to be seen. It is also possible that the EEG effects of neuroleptic drugs, being global, override whatever indigenous patterns exist and thus create the appearance of symmetry.

In a study of mean integrated amplitude (MIA) of 18 depressed psychotics, before and after convulsive therapy, with either bilateral electroconvulsive treatment (ECT) or Indoklon-therapy, d'Elia and Perris found that MIA increased after treatment.[30] Although there were no interhemispheric differences before or after treatment, the authors considered that the dominant hemisphere was more involved in depressive states than the non-dominant one, mainly on the basis of lower MIA variance on the left side and a correlation of depression score with a low L/R ratio. As a low L/R ratio, however, can be reflecting a larger amplitude on the right or nondominant side, and since, as we shall see later, right-sided large amplitude phenomena tend to accompany affective disorders, their conclusion needs reconsideration.

In a subsequent study, d'Elia, et al investigated 28 schizophrenic inpatients treated with penfluridol or thiothixene.[31] Their study confirmed once again that MIA can increase as a result of drug treatment or clinical improvement. Reduction of MIA L/R ratio was found to be the most promising variable in reflecting the effect of treatment. Considering the reversal of L/R ratio[29] seen in psychotic and drug induced states and which we interpreted as signifying abnormal symmetry, such a trend (>L/R) can be seen as indicative of the restoration of normative asymmetry pari passu treatment.

In a study of interhemispheric relationships in terms of neurophysiological, perceptual and electroencephalographic (EEG) data of psychotic patients before and after different types of somatic treatment, Small, et al found that convulsive therapy was associated with improvement in nonverbal task performance but deterioration of verbal skills.[32] Bilateral ECT was associated with more EEG slowing over the dominant hemisphere; right and left unilateral ECT resulting in nondominant hemisphere slowing early in the course of treatment with EEG changes ipsilateral to the side of unilateral ECT developing later. It should be emphasized, however, that there was a persistent increase in the mean energy content (amplitude) of the EEG over the dominant hemisphere regardless of the side of unilateral ECT. This phenomenon can be interpreted in a nonspecific sense as denoting the sensitivity of the dominant hemisphere in reflecting interference with cerebral functioning of any kind—indeed, it might prove a unique index of cerebral disturbance—and claims such as the ones by d'Elia, et al[30,31] mentioned earlier might have to be reconsidered in this light. On the other hand, the role of the nondominant hemisphere in depression is possibly strengthened with additional evidence in view of the EEG findings mentioned above. In this connection it should also be added that the same investigators found that lithium affected visuospatial, i.e. nondominant hemisphere, functions;[32] the implications, considering the effects of lithium on depression, are again strongly suggestive about the significance of the nondominant hemisphere in this respect.

Flor-Henry, after reviewing the published literature, concluded that the evidence so far suggests predominantly unilateral dominant hemisphere neuronal disorganization as associated with the schizophrenic syndrome, and predominantly unilateral nondominant hemisphere dysfunction as associated with the affective psychoses. He also mentions as possibilities bilateral temporal limbic dysfunction associated with schizophrenia and bilateral orbito-fronto limbic dysfunction as possibly associated with affective disorders.[33]

In a later formulation he claims that the evidence suggests that mood states are regulated by orbital and mesial frontal structures bilaterally and, unilaterally, by the nondominant for speech cerebral hemisphere (frontotemporal limbic structures). He also invokes as necessary for his schema of psychopathological manifestations, the principle of active reciprocal interaction between the two hemispheres, whereby anger, euphoria, and paranoid mood are generated when the nondominant hemisphere no longer controls the dominant systems, whereas dysphoric emotions or anxiety are, conversely, generated when the nondominant hemisphere itself is no longer controlled by the dominant one.[34] This principle was previously promulgated, on the basis of empirical evidence involving induced speech phenomena, by Driver, et al, who hypothesized the existence of reciprocal excitation-inhibition processes between the two hemispheres involving speech and, perhaps, responsible for the manifestation of phenomena such as ictal speech automatisms, where the nondominant hemisphere seems to be involved as often as the dominant one.[35]

In an even more speculative vein, Galin put forward the hypothesis that "in normal intact people mental events in the right hemisphere can become disconnected functionally from the left hemisphere (by inhibition of neuronal transmission across the cerebral commissures), and can continue a life of their own. This hypothesis suggests a neurophysiological mechanism for at least some instances of repression and an anatomical locus for the unconscious mental contents."[36] It should be noted, however, that even if one accepts, for heuristic purposes, that such events can take place in normal intact people, this does not by itself offer a ready made model for psychotic patients or psychotic processes. The difficulties encountered by psychoanalytically inclined psychiatrists in applying to psychoses the lessons learned by Freud in studying neuroses, are instructive and should be kept in mind.

In terms of visual evoked potential (VEP) studies one ought to mention Roemer, et al, who investigated possible lateralized hemispheric dysfunction in schizophrenia based on the spatial distribution (12 electrodes) of a measure of VEP wave form stability over time. The authors found that VEP wave form stability was generally lower in all types of schizophrenia in comparison to normals and that VEPs differed more between the hemispheres in schizophrenics and psychotic depressives than in nonpsychotic subjects; furthermore whereas left hemisphere stability was abnormal in schizophrenics it was normal in psychotic depressives. Even in latent schizophrenics VEP stability differences between the hemispheres were greater than normal, with less stability on the left. The authors concluded that their results did provide a direct demonstration of a left hemisphere involvement in schizophrenic dysfunction.[37]

In a subsequent report the same authors tried to determine whether the VEP findings would extend to the auditory (AEP) and somatosensory (SEP) modalities. Indeed, they found that overtly psychotic schizophrenics exhibited lower than normal stability in left hemisphere AEPs. However, no such asymmetry was found for SEP. Thus they concluded that only the AEP results confirm their previous VEP evidence indicating left hemisphere dysfunction in schizophrenics.[38]

Finally, French investigators have been publishing reports confirming many of the findings already mentioned in this section, namely L/R ratio changes in schizophrenics versus normals. The reports suggest the presence of lateralized hyperarousal and interhemispheric dysfunction in schizophrenics.[39]

LATERALITY PATTERNS IN ALCOHOLISM AND SCHIZOPHRENIA

Two questions considered of importance in the development of multivariate patterning techniques for the investigation of neurophysiological processes in psychopathology are (1) whether a model of "normal" EEG structure would apply to psychiatric groups so that comparisons could be made in terms of levels of activity, and (2) whether subgroups and individual subject factor structure could give information on the presence of unique processes. To answer such questions, we have been performing over the last few years analyses of EEG power bands along with other EEG variables of potential significance in a variety of inpatient populations in a psychiatric hospital.[40,41] The variables include EEG power in 2 Hz bands from 0 to 40 Hz, power asymmetry in 2 Hz bands, average evoked response (AER) amplitude, peak latency and amplitude-intensity (A-I) slope, among others. The purpose is to determine the factor structure in these patients versus the normal population employed by Defayolle and Dinnand,[42] as well as to look at the interrelationships between these various measures of CNS activity.

It is hoped that factor structure as well as factor scores may provide the most objective means available at the present time to test hypotheses about basic processes underlying various psychiatric conditions. Using such techniques one can test a number of predictions concerning the EEG asymmetries associated with various subgroups of psychiatric patients, e.g.:[12]

1. As paranoid delusions involve the utilization of verbal-analytic processes, and as such processes have generally been ascribed to the dominant (most often left) cerebral hemisphere, patients with paranoid symptoms would show EEG patterns reflecting activation of the left hemisphere.

2. As affective and hallucinatory symptoms, such as those exhibited by
   hebephrenic and schizo-affective patients, appear to involve holistic or
   nonlinear cognitive styles, and as affective symptoms have been found to
   be associated with right hemisphere functions, patients with such
   symptoms would show EEG patterns reflecting activation of the right
   hemisphere.
3. As, finally, in chronic psychotics of the undifferentiated type, the assumption could be made of a condition suggesting lack of hemispherically
   related dominant behavioral patterns, in such patients EEG patterns would
   reflect symmetry rather than asymmetry.

Additionally such techniques can be used to investigate the relation between type of symptoms and patterns of laterality in psychiatric patients as a
function of clinical change or medication in the hospital, since there is evidence of increased EEG asymmetry following inpatient treatment of schizophrenic patients.[10-11] The purpose of such studies is to explore the
psychophysiologic state in the psychiatric patient by the intercorrelation of
longitudinal data obtained from psychological testing, clinical assessment,
and electrophysiological measurements. What follows is a brief account of
some of the significant facts found so far.

Some AER measures have been recently developed, as already mentioned, which show promise of differentiating between patient groups. One of
these is A-I function, i.e. the change in evoked potential amplitude as a
function of stimulus intensity, which is reported to differentiate psychiatric
groups as well as to change as a function of clinical improvements.[43,44] A-I
slope, amplitude, and the symmetry of the AER amplitude have been shown
to be responsive to alcohol ingestion.[45,46] Lewis, et al found that hemispheric
amplitude differences for the AER tended to disappear following alcohol
ingestion.[47] As both A-I slope and symmetry of the AER are responsive to
alcohol, progressive effects of exposure and withdrawal from alcohol could be
reflected in these measures.

We studied three groups of subjects, including 17 male alcoholic patients
undergoing alcoholic withdrawal, 27 male alcoholic patients who had been
stabilized for three to four weeks after withdrawal, and 30 male volunteers.[13]
Both patient groups were receiving equivalent doses of Antabuse at the time
of recordings. The alcoholics of both groups were receiving 250 mg per day at
the time of the recordings. All control subjects were completely unmedicated.

The left-right asymmetry of AER amplitude, previously reported for
normal subjects,[46,47] was tested by each intensity. The stabilized alcoholics
showed significantly greater left hemisphere amplitudes at the highest flash
intensities. None of the other hemispheric comparisons was significant. When
the left-right differences were considered without regard to direction, the

withdrawal alcoholics showed generally smaller left-right differences than other groups. The withdrawal group had significantly smaller differences, or greater symmetry, than controls at the lowest flash intensity.

Also the withdrawal alcoholics showed a consistent tendency toward lower bilateral amplitude differences at all intensity levels. This would suggest that greater bilateral symmetry accompanies alcohol withdrawal.

Alcohol, of course, like many other drugs, can produce cerebral damage with prolonged exposure or chronic use. Bennett reviewed evidence for cerebral atrophy in alcoholism and found that chronic alcoholics show up to 87 percent incidence of cerebral atrophy, as indicated by the pneumoencephalogram (PEG), with 8 percent showing only cortical atrophy, 44 percent showing only subcortical atrophy with widening of the ventricles, and 48 percent showing both cortical and subcortical atrophy.[48] Alcohol can also produce EEG abnormalities, namely increased 15−30 Hz fast activity and 4−7 Hz slow activity.[48,49] The highest incidence of irreversible EEG abnormalities is found associated with cerebral atrophy, in Wernicke's and Korsakoff's diseases.

Other authors, using visual inspection of the EEG, found in addition widespread fast activity associated with chronic alcoholism.[50−53] Such high frequency abnormalities in the EEGs of chronic alcoholics were found to be significantly related to impaired cognitive performance, symptoms of hallucinosis and DTs, as well as the acute brain syndrome.

Our own findings showed that high frequency EEG activity separated two groups of alcoholics who were matched according to both age and the number of years they reported as having had a drinking problem.[14] They differed however, clinically, insofar that tests indicated severe cognitive impairment in one group and less impairment for the other group. Both groups had increased precentral power in all but the 8−12 Hz band in comparison to age-matched control subjects, but in the high frequency bands, the mean power values appeared systematically ordered from high to low from the impaired alcoholics to unimpaired to controls, especially in the precentral derivations. These significant correlations between high frequency power and cognitive impairment support the hypothesis that frontotemporal high frequency activity may reflect atrophy accompanying prolonged alcohol ingestion.

Another contribution that quantified clinical neurophysiology has made in psychiatric research is in the area of the value of the EEG in psychiatric diagnosis. This has frequently been questioned because of the nonspecificity of EEG findings of different psychiatric groups. For instance, as detailed below, although proposed etiologies, and recognized symptoms, for two conditions as disparate as alcoholism and schizophrenia, have few if any similarities, the EEG findings have been shown to have similar characteristics. These include increased low frequency EEG components and increased power in higher frequency bands.[48-58] An alternative view, one that we investigated, is that even though such findings appear to reinforce the notion of EEG nonspecificity, they may also reflect similar neurophysiological mechanisms underlying apparently diverse psychiatric syndromes.

For this study we compared fifteen chronic nonparanoid patients, between the ages of 19 and 56 with a mean of 37.9 (S.D. 11.9) years, to 15 age-matched male chronic alcoholics who had been withdrawn from alcohol for a minimum of two weeks and stabilized on Antabuse.[15] Fifteen male control subjects were selected, matched to the schizophrenic and alcoholic subjects' ages.

Indeed our findings showed patterns of differences between controls, schizophrenics and alcoholics which support such a hypothesis. Thus, both patient groups showed higher levels of activity in the low frequency (delta and theta) and high frequency (beta 1) bands, compared to controls, in the left frontotemporal area, while the high frequency differences in the right frontotemporal and bilateral centro-occipital bands appear to be primarily between the alcoholics and controls.

As already mentioned, there is some evidence of a relationship between high frequency (beta 2) power and cerebral impairment seen in chronic alcoholism.[14,48,49]

Also, the presence of the high frequency abnormality in the EEGs of chronic alcoholics has been found to be significantly related to impaired cognitive performance, and acute brain syndrome.[52,53] Schizophrenics have been also shown to have more bursts of 18−24 Hz, mainly prefrontal, activity than control subjects, with alcoholics falling in between.[14,15,53-58]

Additional evidence for precentral, and particularly left lateralized, cerebral dysfunction in schizophrenics has been provided through behavioral observation,[59] the EEG,[60] the use of tests designed for localizing brain impairment,[61] and measures of cerebral blood flow rate.[62,63]

Computer analyzed EEGs have generally demonstrated increased amplitude of high frequency and low frequency bands, predominantly over precentral recording sites, similar to our own findings.[55-58,60]

To recapitulate, the differences in high frequency between chronic alcoholics and controls in the frontotemporal derivations would be consistent with the hypothesis that anterior bilateral brain impairment may exist in these patients. This was supported by psychometric tests in these patients, showing marked impairment. As to the data showing elevated high frequency activity in the left precentral derivation in schizophrenics, these are interpreted as indicating the presence of a perhaps similar type of impairment, but lateralized in the left anterior area of the brain.

Research could, through careful analysis of different schizophrenic subgroups, shed some light on the potential mechanisms underlying such differences. As, for instance, symptoms vary considerably among subgroups of schizophrenic patients it would seem important to consider the possibility that different patients may have dysfunctions in different areas of the brain, possibly reflected either in ongoing brain activity or in the reactivity of the brain to stimulation.

Indeed, the category of schizophrenias encompasses a wide variety of symptoms, some of which could be classified as related to left brain dysfunction while others could be classified as being predominantly related to right brain dysfunction. Based on this concept we attempted to determine whether schizophrenic patients who showed either predominantly left or right symptoms, as measured by BPRS scales,[64] distinguished according to factors such as thought disorder and hostility (left side), or anxiety and tension (right side), differed from each other or from a matched control group in terms of EEG and evoked potential asymmetries.[65]

Out of an initial population of 30 schizophrenic patients interviewed, a total of 6 patients showed an unmixed pattern of right hemispheric symptoms and 8 showed left hemispheric symptoms only. These subgroups had mean ages of 32.5 and 26.4, respectively. A group of volunteer subjects from the staff were selected with the same range of age as the schizophrenics (24 to 37; mean = 32).

Power spectral density (PSD) analysis was performed using a Nicolet MED-80 computer. The PSDs were averaged for three epochs in 2 Hz bands from 0 to 30 Hz for all four derivations. The findings were that patients with predominantly left symptoms appear to show larger amplitude of high frequency activity in the left anterior derivation (frontotemporal) than on the right. Patients with right symptoms showed bilateral elevation of amplitude in the high frequency bands. The reverse was true in terms of visual evoked responses, i.e. elevation of right side amplitude in right symptom patients, but no difference in left symptom patients.[65]

Thus, the indications, already mentioned, that the schizophrenic patients may have a left lateralized type of impairment which is reflected by an asymmetry in high frequency bands of the EEG, was found in this study only for patients with left lateralized symptoms. The patient group with predominantly left, or thought-disorder type symptoms, showed a pattern of increased amplitude in the left frontotemporal high frequency activity as compared to the right. This, of course, suggests that thought disorder type of symptoms are closely related to the left frontotemporal areas in schizophrenics. The group with right hemisphere symptoms, on the other hand, showed increased high frequency activity in both frontotemporal derivations, whereas the age-matched controls showed little asymmetry and had less voltage at high frequencies than the patient groups.

In the AER, however, the patients with right symptoms showed significant, but opposite, asymmetries. (R>L). In view of the usual symmetry of visual evoked potentials in normal subjects[66] and the reliability of such measurements,[67,68] any such asymmetry, unless task or input related,[69] must be considered very carefully. Perris showed increased amplitude of AER of the non-dominant hemisphere in depressive patients in comparison to schizophrenic patients.[70] Landau, Buchsbaum, et al, also showed that bipolar patients had higher mean amplitudes in their AERs than either normal subjects or schizophrenics.[71] Finally, Roemer, Shagass, et al demonstrated, in addition to their other findings discussed earlier, that AER instability between the hemispheres is greater in schizophrenics and depressives than in controls.[37] Thus, a reasonable explanation for our findings[65] may be that as the right symptom schizophrenic group was classified on the basis of affective symptoms, many of which could be considered of a reactive nature, it is possible that higher evoked responses of the right hemisphere were in some way reflecting a right-sided hyperreactivity to emotional stimuli, the latter reported also by others.[72]

The results of these recent studies suggest that the symptoms shown by a patient may be reflecting not only different expressions of a single process, but can also be related to the malfunction of different cerebral processes. These processes, as reflected in different patterns of brain activity, might be then best approached through different treatment modalities, specifically targeted on them. The latter is an area that has not even been really touched yet, but the implications are intriguing. Obviously, further research in the meantime on electrophysiological differences among various types of patients, and under various conditions, e.g. during tasks activating the left and right hemisphere respectively, is more than warranted, since our information about the various possible distinguishing patterns of electrophysiological activity in various mental disorders is far from complete.

THE RELATIONSHIP OF CLINICAL TO ELECTROPHYSIOLOGICAL PHENOMENA

The previous sections raise a number of questions regarding the meaning of EEG and AER amplitude differences, either global or interhemispheric, intraindividual or between subjects. In order to conceptualize such differences (Fig. 3-1), we might also visualize a continuum (Fig. 3-2), at the one end of which we encounter large EEG amplitude phenomena of a normative type (e.g., resting), and at the other end, large amplitude phenomena due to pathological causes (e.g., lesions or drug effects). In between, we have the reduced amplitude of task-related functions, and the even more reduced

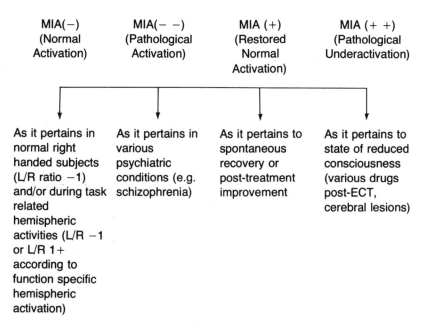

MIA(−) (Normal Activation)	MIA(− −) (Pathological Activation)	MIA (+) (Restored Normal Activation)	MIA (+ +) (Pathological Underactivation)
As it pertains in normal right handed subjects (L/R ratio −1) and/or during task related hemispheric activities (L/R −1 or L/R 1+ according to function specific hemispheric activation)	As it pertains in various psychiatric conditions (e.g. schizophrenia)	As it pertains to spontaneous recovery or post-treatment improvement	As it pertains to state of reduced consciousness (various drugs post-ECT, cerebral lesions)

Fig. 3-1.   Interpretations of MIA changes. MIA = mean integrated amplitude; − = reduction; + = increase; L = left hemisphere; R = right hemisphere.

amplitude seen in dysfunctional states, whether endogenous (psychosis) or drug-induced. Restoration of function, either spontaneous or through treatment, is usually accompanied by increase in amplitude, although beyond a certain point medication can lead to the excessively large amplitude seen at the pathological end of the continuum. It is also, perhaps, fair to say that whereas interhemispheric asymmetry is enhanced during alertness and task-related functions, it tends to be abolished at the ends and in the middle of the continuum, that is, whenever amplitude measures are at their maximum or minimum and when symmetry is the rule rather than the exception.

What all this means is that amplitude measurements can be used as indicators of cerebral efficiency only in relation to their relative position and direction at any particular time. Thus, we need to distinguish between an expected reduction of amplitude, as seen in either hemisphere, when functions appropriate to that hemisphere are performed, and an unexpected one, seen while the subject is ostensibly resting and which, in fact, might signify arousal or activation of a psychotic type. Conversely, an increase of amplitude, especially following an excessive previous reduction of the type mentioned before, might accompany improvement in functioning, when coinciding with clinical

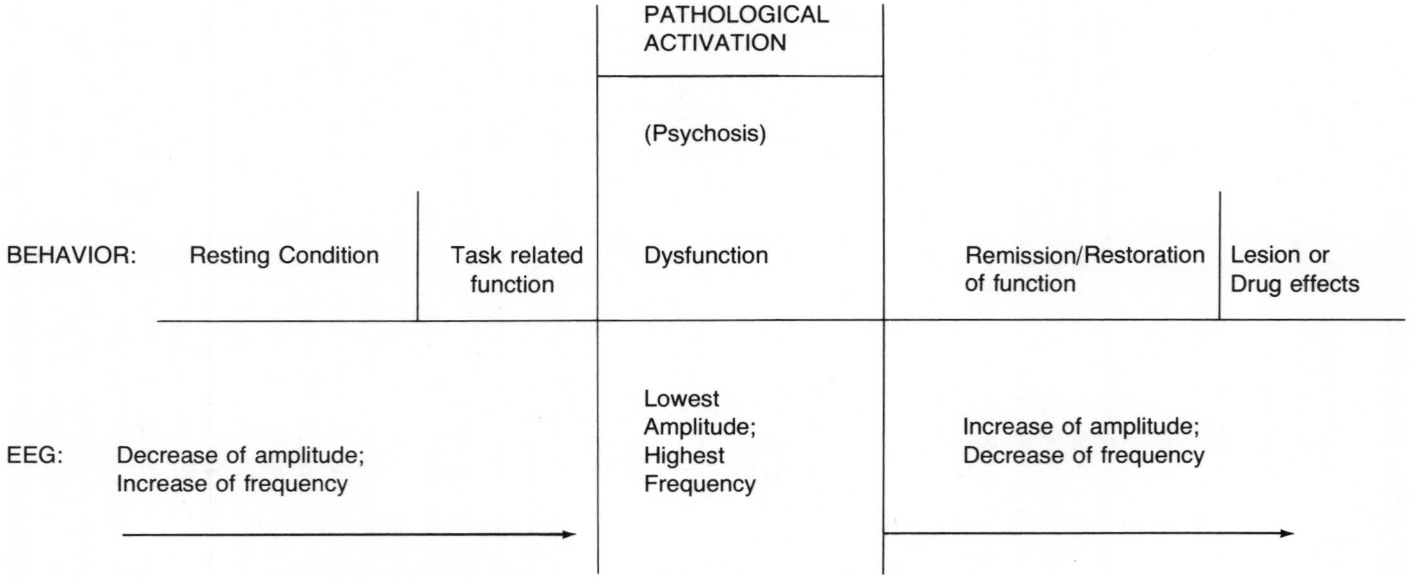

Fig. 3-2. Continuum showing EEG amplitude and frequency changes as they relate to cerebral functioning in normal and pathological conditions.

52

improvement, and thus should not be automatically interpreted as evidence of reduced vigilance.

The inverse relationship between amplitude and frequency, as it usually pertains to nonepileptic EEGs, makes it possible in such a continuum to associate low and high frequencies with large and small amplitudes, respectively. This kind of continuum should, of course, be supplemented by another, more clinico-pathological, schema for the understanding of the inter-hemispheric amplitude and frequency phenomena in terms of cerebral functioning and associated clinical phenomena.

Cerebral dysfunction can be the result of many causes. These can be classified as either physiological or structural (anatomical) in nature. Examples of the former are dysfunctions produced by drugs; of the latter, dysfunctions produced by anatomical lesions. Sometimes a certain overlapping is present, as for instance, when a head injury causes epilepsy: the observed results are due in part to the structural lesion and in part to the physiological disturbance associated with seizures. It is also, perhaps, true to say that whereas physiological dysfunctions are of a limited duration or occur episodically, structural dysfunctions tend to be longer lasting if not permanent. However it is produced, a cerebral dysfunction is characterized by at least three principles responsible for the observed phenomena. As Figure 3-3 shows, these are: the principle of cerebral deficit (e.g., contralateral paralysis following motor cortex lesions); the principle of disinhibition (e.g., contralateral spasm also ensuing upon such lesions); and the principle of adaptation (e.g., restoration of spared function, assisted by the whole organism, in the phase of rehabilitation). Difficulties arise when one attempts to transpose such a schema from the concrete area of motor cortex lesions and their sequels to the much more complex and elusive area of association cortex. However, and despite the fact that any such attempt at this stage of our knowledge is bound to be incomplete and in many ways arbitrary, yet it has to be made, even if for heuristic purposes alone, considering the confusing and apparently contradictory claims of the literature in the area of cerebral lateralization and behavior. Without the help of these principles, i.e. deficit, disinhibition and adaptation-compensation, it is difficult to reconcile claims incriminating either hemisphere for similar, if not identical, symptoms.

In the formulation of such postulates, one must also employ some crucial assumptions (Fig. 3-4). These are, the assumption that in the dominant hemisphere phenomena the crucial dysfunction involves time-sequencing and pacing of mental events, impairment of which leads to inability to hold or defer, with resulting explosive simultaneity of behavioral output events, and, in regard to nondominant hemisphere phenomena, the assumption that the crucial dysfunction here involves the spatial framing of mental events, impairment of which leads to a loss of perspective, with resulting implosive effects on mood.

Non-Dominant Hemisphere
Anatomical and/or Physiological
Dysfunction

DEFICIT PHENOMENA

Contralateral
Hemiplegia

Contralateral
Hemianesthesia

Proprioceptive deficits

Visuo-Spatial
Orientation deficits

Self-Space disorientation
(Body-image)

DISINHIBITION
PHENOMENA

Contralateral
Twitchings and
Convulsions

Contralateral
Hypersensitivity

(Belle indifference;
disassociation
phenomena)

(Hallucination/illusion)
(Delusions)

(Mood Lability)
(Depression)

ADAPTATION-
COMPENSATION
PHENOMENA

DISINHIBITION
PHENOMENA

Contralateral
Twitchings and
Convulsions

Contralateral
Hypersensitivity

Speech compensatory
symptoms (speech
automatisms)

(Paranoid thought)
(Delusions)

(Confabulation)

(Aggression Impulse
dyscontrol)
(catastrophic reaction
including depression or
grandiosity)

Dominant Hemisphere
Anatomical and/or Physiological
Dysfunction

DEFICIT PHENOMENA

Contralateral
Hemiplegia

Contralateral
Hemianesthesia

Aphasia and other
Speech disorders

Thought Disorder

Agnosias
Memory deficits
Dyxlexias

Learning deficits

UNCONSCIOUSNESS

SOMATAGNOSIA
NOSAGNOSIA

HEURISTIC CATEGORIES	DOMINANT HEMISPHERE PHENOMENA	NON-DOMINANT HEMISPHERE PHENOMENA
Assumed Normal Function Mode	Time-sequencing and pacing of symbolic input-output	Framing and ordering of visuo-spatial perceptions
Dysfunctional Principles (Anatomical and/or Physiological)	Deficit Disinhibition Compensation/Adaptation	Deficit Disinhibition Compensation/Adaptation
Assumed Dysfunctional Mode	Impaired time-sequencing and pacing of symbolic input-output	Impaired framing and ordering of visuo-spatial perceptions
Process description of dysfunction	Inability to defer or hold and process input-output in terms of comparison and alternative choices	Inability to relate parts to whole and vice versa; to form perspective; to map
Behavioral description of dysfunction	"Explosiveness" or simultaneity of processes	"Implosiveness" or diffusion of processes

CLINICAL INSTANCES

Epilepsy	Impulse dyscontrol (violent aggression)	Depressive episodes; hallucinations, illusions
Schizophrenia	Paranoid thought disorder (violent aggression)	Depressive episodes; hallucinations, illusions
Affective Disorder	Hypomanic behavior (violent aggression)	Depressive episodes

Fig. 3-4. Cerebral dysfunction and associated phenomena: heuristic and clinical assumptions.

Fig. 3-3.(Opposite page.) Cerebral dysfunction and associated phenomena: tentative classification of underlying principles. Arrows indicate phenomena that, regardless of hemispheric origin, may also be global adaptation-compensation phenomena.

55

Such formulations, tentative or otherwise, need to be translated into testable hypotheses and then put to the rigors of experimental verification before becoming acceptable coinage, useful for therapeutic practice. As shown earlier in the chapter, there already is evidence supporting a number of them. However, the bulk of the work and the necessary proof still lie ahead, beckoning future endeavors. A useful reminder of this is offered by the example of the pathogenesis of aggressive outbursts.[73] Either hemisphere can be implicated in such an outburst, if its functions are interfered with: the dominant one, because of its role in learned behavior, especially verbal, and thus its significance in catastrophic reactions; and the nondominant one, because of its role in affect, and thus its significance in mood instability. Research along these lines might identify other similar mechanisms, operating, according to the case in question, through the one or the other hemisphere.

REFERENCES

1. Serafetinides EA, Hoare RD, Driver MV: A modification of the intracarotid sodium amylobarbitone test. Lancet 1:249–250, 1964
2. Serafetinides EA, Hoare RD, Driver MV: Intracarotid sodium amytal and cerebral dominance for speech and consciousness. Brain 88:107–130, 1965
3. Serafetinides EA, Hoare RD, Driver MV: EEG patterns induced by intracarotid injection of sodium amytal. Electroenceph Clin Neurophysiol 18:170–175, 1965
4. Serafetinides EA: Aggressiveness in temporal lobe epileptics and its relation to cerebral dysfunction and environmental factors. Epilepsia 6:33–42, 1965
5. Serafetinides EA: The significance of the temporal lobes and of hemispheric dominance in the production of LSD-25 symptomatology in man. Neuropsychologia 3:69–79, 1965
6. Serafetinides EA: Brain laterality: New functional aspects, in Kourilsky R and Grapin P (eds): Main droite et main gauche, Presses Universitaires de France, Paris, 1968
7. Serafetinides EA, Walter RD, Cherlow D: Amnestic confusional phenomena, hippocampal stimulation and laterality factors, in Isaacson RL and Pribram KH (eds): Hippocampus, vol 2. New York, Plenum, 1975, pp 363–375
8. Rausch R, Serafetinides EA, Crandall PH: Olfactory memory in patients with anterior temporal lobectomy. Cortex 13:445–452, 1977
9. Serafetinides EA, Walter RD: Induced amnestic confusional phenomena: pathology and lateralization. J Nerv Ment Dis 166:661–662, 1978
10. Serafetinides EA: Laterality and voltage in the EEG of psychiatric patients. Dis Nerv Syst 33:622–623, 1972
11. Serafetinides EA: Voltage laterality in the EEG of psychiatric patients. Dis Nerv Syst 34:190–191, 1973
12. Serafetinides EA: Quantitative electroencephalography in psychiatric research,

in Deniker P, Radouco-Thomas C, and Villeneuve A (eds): Neuro-psychopharmacology, Proceedings of the 10th Congress of the Collegium International Neuropsychopharmacologium (vol. 2). Oxford/N.Y., Pergamon Press, 1978

13. Coger RW, Dymond AM, Serafetinides EA, et al: Alcoholism: Averaged visual evoked response amplitude-intensity slope and symmetry in withdrawal. Biol Psychiat 11:435−443, 1976

14. Coger RW, Dymond AM, Serafetinides EA: EEG signs of brain impairment in alcoholism. Biol Psychiat 13:729−739, 1978

15. Coger RW, Dymond AM, Serafetinides EA: EEG similarities between chronic alcoholics and chronic, non-paranoid schizophrenics. Arch Gen Psychiat 36:91−94, 1979

16. Gazzaniga MS: The Bisected Brain. New York, Appleton-Century-Crofts, 1970

17. Gazzaniga MS, LeDoux JE: The Integrated Mind. New York, Plenum Press, 1978

18. Kinsbourne MD, Lynn Smith W (eds): Hemispheric Disconnection and Cerebral Function. Springfield, C.C. Thomas, 1974

19. TenHouten WD, Kaplan CD: Science and its Minor Image. New York, Harper and Row, 1973

20. Dimond SJ, Baumont J (eds): Hemisphere function in the Human Brain. New York, J Wiley & Sons, 1974

21. Desmedt JE (ed): Language and Hemispheric Specialization in Man: Cerebral Event-Related Potentials. New York, S Karger, 1977

22. Weinstein EA, Friedland RP (eds): Hemi-Inattention and Hemisphere Specialization. New York, Raven Press, 1977

23. Dimond SJ, Blizard DA (eds): Evolution and Lateralization of the Brain. New York, N.Y. Academy of Sciences, 1977

24. Harnard S, Doty RW, Goldstein, L, Jaynes J, Krauthamer G (eds): Lateralization in the Nervous System. New York, Academic Press, 1977

25. Shagass C: An electrophysiological view of schizophrenia. Biol Psychiat 11:3−30, 1976

26. Itil T: Qualitative and quantitative EEG findings in schizophrenia. Schizophrenia Bulletin 3:61−79, 1977

27. Giannitrapani D, Kayton L: Schizophrenia and EEG spectral analysis. Electroenceph Clin Neurophysiol 36:377−386, 1974

28. Sugarman AA, Goldstein L, Marjerrison G, et al: Recent research in EEG amplitude analysis. Dis Nerv Syst 34:162−166, 1973

29. Goldstein L, Stoltzfus NW: Psychoactive drug-induced changes of interhemispheric EEG amplitude relationship, in Agents and Actions, vol 3. No. 2 Birkhäser Verlag, Basel, 1973 pp. 124−132

30. d'Elia G, Perris C: Cerebral functional dominance and depression. Acta Psychiat Scand 49:191−197, 1973

31. d'Elia G, Jacobsson L, Von Knorring L, et al: Changes in psychophathology in relation to EEG variables and visual averaged evoked responses (VAER) in schizophrenic patients treated with penfluridol or thithixene. Acta Psychiat Scand 55:309−318, 1977

32. Small IF, Small JC, Milstein V, et al: Interhemispheric relationships with somatic therapy. Dis Nerv Syst 34:170−177, 1973

33. Flor-Henry P: Psychiatric syndromes considered as manisfestations of lateralized temporal-limbic dysfunction, in surgical approaches in psychiatry, in Laitinen LV, Livingston KE (eds): Surgical Approaches in Psychiatry, Baltimore, University Park Press, 1973, pp 22−26

34. Flor-Henry P: On certain aspects of the localization of the cerebral systems regulating and determining emotion. Biol Psychiat 14:677−698, 1979

35. Driver, MV, Falconer, MA, Serafetinides EA: Ictal speech automatism reproduced by activation procedures. Neurology 14:455−463, 1964

36. Galin D: Implications for psychiatry of left and right cerebral specialization. Arch Gen Psychiat 31:572−583, 1974

37. Roemer RA, Shagass C, Straumanis JJ, et al: Pattern evoked potential measurements suggesting lateralized hemispheric dysfunction in chronic schizophrenics. Biol Psychiat 13:185−202, 1978

38. Roemer RA, Shagass C, Straumanis JJ, et al: Somatosensory and auditory evoked potential studies of functional differences between the cerebral hemispheres in psychosis. Biol Psychiat 14:354−373, 1979

39. Etevenon P, Pidoux B, Rioux P, et al: Intra-and interhemispheric EEG differences quantified by spectral analysis. Acta Psychiat Scand 60:57−68, 1979

40. Coger RW, Dymond AM, Serafetinides EA, et al: Factor analytic relations among EEG variables in an alcoholic population. Proc San Diego Biomed Symp 14:67−70, 1975

41. Coger RW, Dymond AM, Serafetinides EA: Classification of psychiatric patients with factor analytic EEG variables. Proc San Diego Biomed Symp 15:279−284, 1976

42. Defayolle M, Dinand JP: Application of factor analysis to the study of EEG structure. Electroenceph Clin Neurophysiol 36:319−322, 1974

43. Buchsbaum M, Silverman J: Stimulus intensity control and the cortical evoked response. Psychosom Med 30:12−22, 1968

44. Singer M, Borge G, Almond R, et al: Correlation between phenothiazine administration, clinical course and perceptual (neurophysiological) measures. Clin Res 17:133, 1969

45. Spilker B, Callaway E: Effects of drugs on "augmenting—reducing" in averaged visual evoked responses in man. Psychopharmacologia 15:116−124, 1969

46. Rhodes LE, Obitz FW, Creel D: Effects of alcohol and task on hemispheric asymmetry of visually evoked potentials in man. Electroenceph Clin Neurophysiol 38:561−568, 1975

47. Lewis EG, Dustman RE, Beck EC: The effect of alcohol on visual and somatosensory evoked responses. Electroenceph Clin Neurophysiol 28:202−205, 1970

48. Bennett AE: Diagnosis of intermediate stage of alcohol brain disease. J.A.M.A. 172:1143−1146, 1960

49. Bennett AE, Mowery GL, Fort JT: Brain damage from chronic alcoholism: The diagnosis of intermediate stage of alcoholic brain disease. Am J Psychiat 116:705−711, 1960

50. Bennett AE, Doi LT, Mowery GL: The value of electroencephalography in alcoholism. J Nerv Ment Dis 124:27−32, 1956

51. Funkhouser JB, Nagler B, Walke ND: The electroencephalogram of chronic alcoholism. Southern Med J 46:423−428, 1953

52. Kennard MA, Bueding E, Wortis SB: Some biochemical and electroencephalographic changes in delerium tremens. Quart J Stud Alc 6:4−14, 1945

53. Lester BK, Edwards RJ: EEG fast activity in schizophrenic and control subjects. Int J Neuropsychiat 2:145−156, 1966

54. Serafetinides EA, Willis D, Clark ML: EEG dose-response relationships of chlorpromazine in chronic schizophrenia. Biol Psychiat 4:251−256, 1972

55. Serafetinides EA: EEG studies in chronic alcoholism. Electroenceph Clin Neurophysiol 33:237, 1972

56. Lifshitz K, Gradijan J: Spectral evaluation of the electroencephalogram: Power and variability in chronic schizophrenics and control subjects. Psychophysiol 11:479−490, 1974

57. Simeon J, Itil TM: Computerized electroencephalogram: A model for understanding the brain function in childhood psychosis and its treatment. J Autism Child Schizo 5:247−265, 1975

58. Itil TM, Hau W, Saletu B, et al: Computer EEG and auditory evoked potential investigations in children at high risk for schizophrenia. Am J Psychiat 131:892−900, 1974

59. Flor-Henry P: Ictal and interictal psychiatric manifestations in epilepsy: Specific or non-specific? Epilepsia 13:773−783, 1972

60. Flor-Henry P, Koles ZJ, Bo-Lassen, P, et al: Studies of the functional psychoses: Power spectral EEG analysis. I.C.R.S. Med Sci 3:87, 1975a, (abstr)

61. Flor-Henry, P, Yeudall LT, Stefanyk W, et al: The neuropsychological correlates of the functional psychoses. I.C.R.S. Med Sci 3:34, 1975b, (abstr)

62. Ingvar DH, Franzen G: Abnormalities of cerebral blood flow distribution on patients with chronic schizophrenia. Acta Psychiat Scand 50:425−462, 1974

63. Franzen G, Ingvar DH: Absence of activation in frontal structures during psychological testing of chronic schizophrenics. J Neuro Neurosurg Psychiat 38:1027−1032, 1975

64. Overall JE, Gorham DR: The brief psychiatric rating scale. Psychol Rep 10:799−812, 1962

65. Serafetinides EA, Coger RW, Martin J, et al: Schizophrenic symptomatology and cerebral dominance patterns: A comparison of EEG, AER and BPRS measures. Comp Psychiat (In Press)

66. Harmony T, Ricardo J, Otero G, et al: Symmetry of the visual evoked potential in normal subjects. Electrencephal Clin Neurophysiol 35:237−240, 1973

67. Dustman RE, Beck EC: Long-term stability of visually evoked potentials in man. Science 142:1480−1481, 1963

68. Stark LH, Norton JC: The relative reliability of average evoked response parameters. Psychophysiol 11:600−602, 1974

69. Callaway E: AEP Asymmetry and other individual differences in cortical specialization, in Callaway E (ed): Brain electrical potentials and individual differences. New York, Grune and Stratton, 1975, pp 96−111

70. Perris C: Averaged evoked responses (AER) in patients with affective disorders.

Acta Psychiat Scand, Suppl. 255:89−98, 1974

71. Landau SG, Buchsbaum MS, Carpenter W, et al: Schizophrenia and stimulus intensity control. Arch Gen Psychiat 32:1239−1245, 1975

72. Seliger HH, Biggley WH, Hamman JP: Right hemisphere lateralization for emotion in the human brain: Interactions with cognition. Science 190:286−288, 1975

73. Serafetinides EA: Epilepsy, cerebral dominance and behavior, in Girgis M (ed): Limbic Epilepsy and the Dyscontrol Syndrome. Amsterdam, Elsevier/North Holland (in press)

PART II

Practical and Theoretical Themes

Edward Geller

Introduction

)

The attitude of many mental health practitioners toward biobehavioral drug research may be seen as ranging from ambiguous to paradoxical. Clinicians freely acknowledge the revolution in mental health care that has taken place in the last few decades by writing prescriptions at a pace that makes tranquillizers of all kinds among the most commonly prescribed class of drug today. At the same time, many of these clinicians hold to the opinion that little advance has been made in understanding the neurobiology of mental abnormality. This widely held belief stems from the lack of a comprehensive hypothesis that can easily be seen to offer a rational guide to the design and use of therapeutic agents. Thus, treatments that were perhaps initially developed on an empirical, ad hoc, basis are still widely held as having no firm understanding behind them. That this is an incorrect conception is admirably documented in the chapters of this section, where even a casual reading shows that our increasing understanding of synaptic events is providing a foundation for the actions of psychoactive drugs. It seems inescapably apparent that the actions of these drugs, desirable or not, are deeply involved with synaptic transmission, particularly with synaptic receptor activity.

However, the use and development of psychoactive drugs has provided a major tool for use in the basic research that has led to this greater understanding of the synapse. Specific drugs have been found to have definite biochemical actions at the synapse, some inhibiting enzymes involved in neurotransmitter synthesis, some antagonizing neurotransmitter action at the postsynaptic membrane, some interfering with reuptake systems at presynaptic sites, and some, on the contrary, mimicking the actions of transmitters by stimulating postsynaptic receptors.

The development of these drugs has allowed the identification of receptors in physically isolated membrane receptors from nerve tissue, and has facilitated the study of their properties. Thus, along with the α and β-noradrenergic receptors that have been previously well studied in the peripheral nervous system, receptors for dopamine (at least two), serotonin, and acetylcholine (at least two) have been found in the CNS. In addition, less well studied receptors for peptides, amino acids, steroids, and a group of receptors whose endogenous ligands are not definitely known, but which react with drugs such as the benzodiazapines, have now been identified.

In a similar manner, study of the neuroendocrine effects of psychoactive drugs has contributed much to the understanding of central control mechanisms for release of hormones such as prolactin, TSH, and ACTH, and to a realization of the importance of neurotransmitters in the process. Also, attempts to understand the mechanism of action of lithium have led to advances in the knowledge of transport across neuronal membranes and ion effects at the membrane surface.

The use of psychoactive drugs has thus become a potent tool in basic research and has provided a more precise probe into CNS action, pointing the way to future research.

But basic research has also provided the means to search for and evaluate new drugs. Repeatedly, close correlations have been found between the antischizophrenic action of drugs and the extent to which they compete with the binding of haloperidol to brain membrane preparations. Because haloperidol and dopamine compete for the same receptor sites, strong support is therefore available for a dopamine theory of schizophrenia. Furthermore, the discovery that many dopamine receptors were coupled to an adenylyl cyclase supported a possible role for the dopamine receptor in schizophrenia, since it was soon discovered that the usual α- and β-noradrenergic antagonists had little effect on dopamine-stimulated cyclase, whereas most antipsychotic drugs were potent inhibitors. Continued research in this direction then led to the discovery of a class of dopamine receptors apparently not coupled to adenylyl cyclase. These receptors are found in the hypothalamus where they are involved in the tonic inhibition of prolactin release from the pituitary, and, of particular interest, in the dopaminergic systems of the substantia nigra and of the striatum. Destruction of dopamine nerve endings in the substantia nigra with 6-hydroxydopamine does not alter the activity of the dopamine-sensitive cyclase, while destruction of cell bodies in the striatum with kainic acid produces a substantial decrease in dopamine-sensitive cyclase with little effect on dopamine content. Thus, a class of receptors in the nigra and striatum, felt to be identical to the autoreceptors on dopamine cell bodies previously described, seems not to be associated with cyclase stimulation. The relation, in these anatomical areas, of dopamine to Parkinson's Disease and to tranquilizer-associated Tardive Dyskinesia makes these findings particularly intriguing.

Until recently, research such as that described in general terms above has been based on the assumption of relative constancy of receptor activity. It is now clear that such an assumption is incorrect and that hypo- and hyper-responsivity can be readily demonstrated in many neurotransmitter receptor systems, both at the biochemical and at the behavioral level. These activity changes have been traced to alterations in the number of receptor sites on the postsynaptic membrane, and inhibitors of protein synthesis have been demonstrated to interfere with these changes. The major factor determining the number of receptors seems to be the degree of stimulation of the postsynaptic membrane by transmitter or agonist molecules leading to a kind of feedback-controlled decrease, or subsensitivity, when overstimulated and, conversely, to an increased number, or supersensitivity, when understimulated or inhibited by transmitter antagonists. The rate at which receptor changes can take place is a particularly pertinent question. Single doses of neuroleptic drugs can be demonstrated to elicit supersensitivity in dopaminergic systems and the response can be seen in days. Indeed, in some systems such receptor modulation can be seen within hours. Such rapid response leads to the hypothesis that we are observing a manifestation of homeostatic mechanisms participating in synaptic efficiency and perhaps related to such processes as learning and memory. The interrelation of research and practice as it pertains to psychopharmacology has therefore brought us to the present position where practical approaches to fundamental brain processes are available, surely a long way from purely empirically based treatment.

Ching-Piao Chien

4
Psychopharmacology

Although a wide variety of treatment modalities, somatic as well as nonsomatic, have been developed and introduced in the treatment of mental patients during the last two centuries, none has brought about such significant and unparalleled change as modern psychopharmacotherapy. Since the introduction of chlorpromazine, a first prototype of antipsychotic drugs in the early 1950s, a revolutionary change has occurred in the total mental hospital picture all over the world. Prior to the chlorpromazine era, somatic treatment, such as hydrotherapy, electroshock treatment (EST), insulin shock treatment (IST), prolonged sleep therapy (PST), and even the controversial lobotomy, along with many other nonsomatic treatments, such as morale therapy, individual or group psychotherapy, recreational and milieu therapies, etc., could not prevent the steady increase in the number of patients in mental hospitals. In the United States this number exceeded half a million by the mid-1950s. These mental patients occupied more than half of the total American hospital beds, and the increase would have continued were it not for the large scale usage of chlorpromazine in 1955. Most of these patients were within the wage-earning age bracket, constituting an enormous loss to society in terms of both human and economic resources. Ever since 1955 there has been a substantial, steady decrease in the resident population of mental hospitals, leading in 1979 to an all-time low of fewer than 180,000 patients. Although other factors, such as more progressive mental health laws, psychiatric rehabilitation, community residential programs, and day hospitals have played additional roles, it is commonly accepted that the availability of psychopharmacotherapy has been the major determinant for such a steady change over the last two decades.

    The availability of antidepressant drugs and antianxiety agents since the

67

late 1950s has also made it possible for the family physician to treat many patients in the community who would otherwise have been neglected, or sent to the state hospital. In the late 1960s in the United States, the availability of lithium for the management of the tragic manic-depressive psychosis further prevented incarceration in mental institutions of cyclic affective disorder patients.

SCIENCE OR FAD?

As evidenced by magnetism practiced by mesmerists in the 19th century, there have been in psychiatry several treatment modalities initially accepted with great enthusiasm but which eventually faded away. History has witnessed in the last two centuries the waxing and waning of many such treatment modalities. Without exception, psychotropic drugs were called "chemical straightjackets" and were viewed as another fad by some skeptical psychiatric workers. This view is somewhat reinforced by the current status of chronic schizophrenics who have been on many years of psychotropic drugs but still cannot completely support themselves within the community. In contrast to the initial explosive impact of the phenothiazines on the mental hospital picture, the undesirable scene of chronic mentally ill patients in the slum of the metropolitan city, particularly after the mass deinstitutionalization in the early 1970s, is often connected to the failure of drug treatment, rather than the failure of a total social supportive system.

With the well publicized tardive dyskinesia, a long term neurological side effect from antipsychotic drugs, a wave of pessimism and disillusionment on the current and future role of psychotropic drug treatment began to spread, together with the belief that psychopharmacotherapy is just another fad that will follow the fate of hydrotherapy or insulin shock treatment. Is psychopharmacotherapy really a haphazard practice? Will it fade away because of a lack of theoretical and scientific foundations? To answer these questions, it will be helpful to review the evolutional process of psychopharmacology, the backbone of modern psychotropic drug therapy, within the context of the disciplines involved, and the role it plays in various organizations and programs. One can then have a much better idea of the degree of its validity and durability as a branch of biobehavioral science.

EVOLUTION OF PSYCHOPHARMACOLOGY

As with other medicinal agents, some of the psychotropic drugs were discovered by accident. However, the evolution of psychopharmacological drugs in the last quarter century did not occur merely by sheer luck. Since the effect of psychopharmacotherapy on human behavior is considered to be a complex pharmacophysiological-personality interaction, the disciplines involved in psychopharmacology include psychiatry, pharmacology, physiology, biochemistry, psychology, sociology and anthropology, among others. The Kefauver-Harris Amendment of the Drug Act in 1962 (P.L. 87–781, Oct. 10) stipulated that any prescribed drug marketed in the U.S. should prove its safety and efficacy with scientific data satisfactory to the expert review committee of the Food and Drug Administration. New drugs, both on the market and under clinical investigation, are also regulated by this drug act. The drug inserts or advertisements should contain only facts which have been proven to be truthful and valid. The impact of such an act has made psychopharmacology, as well as clinical pharmacology in other medical specialities, an active branch of science not only in industry but also in academia. The continuous grant support from the psychopharmacology research branch of the National Institute of Mental Health, and also a sizeable funding from the drug industries to the clinicians engaged in early clinical drug evaluation, have vitalized the scientific enterprise of psychopharmacology with thousands of workers representing many disciplines. There have been more than 10,000 papers published already, ranging in scope from the molecular action of the psychotropic drugs on specific enzyme systems to their clinical efficacy in various types of illness. Several textbooks of psychopharmacology have appeared and have been used by medical students, residents, psychiatrists, and even by many paramedical professionals working in the mental health field. Articles in psychopharmacology are ubiquitous in many psychiatric journals. There are also several professional journals exclusively for psychopharmacology studies. An International Reference Center on Psychotropic Drugs was established in the Psychopharmacology Research Branch of the National Institute of Mental Health to promote informational exchanges. The widely distributed Psychopharmacology Bulletin is one of the services provided by this center. Courses in psychopharmacology have been incorporated into the curriculum of medical schools, as well as in residency programs. Periodical seminars, lectures, and workshops in psychopharmacology have become one of the most important activities in the required continuing medical education (CME) program. The American College of Neuropsychopharmacology and The Collegium Internationale Neuropsychopharmacologicum (CINP) are two scientific organizations devoted to the progress of basic and clinical psychopharmacology at the national and international levels. Due to the high quality of the scientific presentations and the high calibre scientists with a track record of achievement as members, these organizations are among the most prestigious of professional scientific organizations. The popular New Clinical Drug Evaluation Unit Program (NCDEU) of NIMH, originally conceived by Gerald Klerman when he was in NIMH, provides a harmonious working atmosphere for workers from governmental agencies, pharmaceutical industries and academia. This program has expedited the standardization of research methodology and evaluation tools in new drug research, not only in the United States but also in many other countries.

The screening procedure, evaluation, and effort to prove the valid efficacy of a psychotropic drug for certain indications appear to be more stringent than those required for nonpharmacological treatment. It is ironic that psychotherapy, another popular treatment modality in the United States has not been subjected to a strict governmental regulation to prove its safety and efficacy as is the case for psychotropic drugs by the Kefauver-Harris Amendment. This is noteworthy when there are many psychotherapists with various training backgrounds practicing therapy in various settings. At a conservative estimate, the money involved in the psychotherapy industry is approximately $500,000,000 annually, if the time of psychiatrists, clinical psychologists, social workers, marriage counselors and others in psychotherapy is taken into account. It therefore seems reasonable to estimate that the size of the psychotherapy industry is at least of an order of magnitude comparable to that of the pharmacotherapy industry.[1] It is hoped that more research be carried out in nonpharmacotherapies at the level of similar sophistication, as seen in the field of psychopharmacology. Only when this has been accomplished can a comprehensive, rational and economical treatment plan be made for our clients.

FROM RESEARCH TO CLINICAL PRACTICE

The achievements of researchers from various disciplines in psychopharmacology over the last quarter century are truly formidable. The information and insights generated in this short period probably surpass those established in the last centuries. These include findings on the molecular structure of neurohormones and neurotransmitters; synapses and receptors; chemical pathways in the brain; basic neuropharmacology and pharmacokinetics; personality and psychosocial factors in the drug treatment outcome; rational and irrational drug treatment according to valid data; therapeutic window; the relative role of drug treatment with psychotherapy; side effects, mechanism and treatment, etc. In this chapter, only the classic examples and studies which are closely related to psychiatric practice will be depicted due to the limitation of space.

Molecular Structure

Molecular structure was demonstrated to explain the antipsychotic property of several psychotropic drugs, especially phenothiazine derivatives. It is generally agreed that all antipsychotic drugs now available in the market exert their therapeutic effects by blocking the dopamine receptors in the CNS, particularly in the mesolimbic system. Elevation of plasma prolactin and manifestation of extrapyramidal symptoms are two well known concomitant phenomena associated with the blocking of dopamine receptors at tuberoinfundibular and nigrostriatal nuclei. Snyder and his coworkers have elegantly demonstrated the resemblance of dopamine molecular structure to part of some phenothiazine structures. The structural resemblance of these two agents can explain why phenothiazines can physically fit and block the dopamine receptors. As shown in Figure 4-1, the side chain of phenothiazines tilts toward the A ring rather than being extended symmetrically between the A and C rings. Such conformations of phenothiazines correspond impressively to the amine and benzene rings of dopamine and indeed can be superimposed.[2-4] Feinberg and Snyder used molecular modeling and computer calculations to predict the antipsychotic potency of various phenothiazines which were consistent in general with the clinical experience. Thus, more potent agents can be designed if we can mimic the dopamine molecular conformation more accurately.

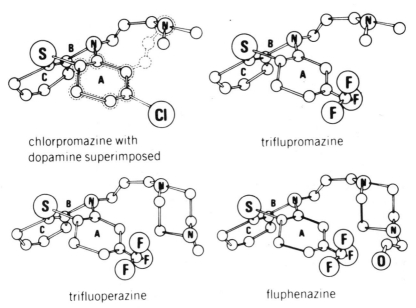

chlorpromazine with
dopamine superimposed

triflupromazine

trifluoperazine

fluphenazine

Fig. 4-1. Phenothiazines with the side chain "tilted" toward the A Ring. From Snyder SH: The dopamine hypothesis of schizophrenia: Focus on the dopamine receptor. Am J Psychiatry 133:199, 1976. Copyright 1976, American Psychiatric Association. (Reproduced with permission.)

Synapses and Receptors

The recent development of synaptology—a discipline involved in the function and mechanism of synapses, the cell membrane, receptors and the mode of neurotransmitter release, reuptake and breakdown, and the metabolic enzymes involved—has increased our understanding of how a chemical agent can affect the CNS at synaptic levels and how the manipulation of synaptic function can affect the behavior. Studies of agonists and antagonists for specific receptors have been actively carried out in the field of behavioral neurology. Tardive dyskinesia and parkinsonism are two major syndromes well studied in connection to dopamine receptors. Idiopathic parkinsonism was assumed to be associated with understimulation of postsynaptic dopamine receptors. This hypothesis derived from the following facts: (1) biochemical analysis of postmortem parkinsonian brain tissue revealed abnormally low levels of dopamine and tyrosine hydroxylase in the caudate nucleus and other regions of the neostriatum, the areas dominated by dopaminergic neurons; (2) morphological analysis revealed cell loss from the substantia nigra, the site of origin of the dopaminergic nigro-striatal system. These findings resulted in the development of a new pharmacological treatment which used the precursor of dopamine—L-Dopa—to correct the insufficient activity of dopamine at the synaptic levels. L-Dopa was used instead of dopamine because the latter would not pass the blood brain barrier. The neuroleptic-induced parkinsonism is clinically identical with idiopathic parkinsonism. This could be well explained by the fact that neuroleptic drugs block the postsynaptic dopamine receptors leading to insufficient dopaminergic activity at postsynaptic neurons, a pathophysiology similar to that of idiopathic parkinsonism. In contrast to the latter, however, there is also an increase of dopamine at the presynaptic neurons. This is well evidenced by the increase of urinary homovanillic acid (HVA), a major metabolite formed during the breakdown of dopamine in the brain. Therefore, one can readily make a differential diagnosis between neuroleptic-induced parkinsonism and idiopathic parkinsonism since the former has high urinary HVA while the latter has low HVA. The increased dopamine at presynaptic neurons is not merely due to the mechanical blockade of postsynaptic dopamine receptors by the neuroleptics; it is also due to the receptor feedback mechanism. The postsynaptic neurons sound an alarm through the feedback reflex to the presynaptic neurons calling for more dopamine when the neuroleptic blockade deprives the postsynaptic receptors. By the same token, when the postsynaptic receptors are flooded by excessive dopamine or its agonists, feedback reflex from the postsynaptic neurons inhibits the production of dopamine at the presynaptic level. Thus, homeostasis of synapses is maintained. It is now postulated that not only postsynaptic receptors but also autoreceptors and presynaptic receptors are involved in this delicate feedback mechanism.[5]

Tardive dyskinesia, a well publicized side effect from long-term usage of neuroleptics, is presumed to be characterized by hypersensitized postsynaptic dopamine receptors. This is similar to the classic "denervation supersensitivity", as described by Cannon and Rosenbleuth in 1949.[6] They showed that the sensitivity of a neuronal receptor is increased when the supply of transmitter is reduced by interruption of afferents. Several studies have been reported in the 1970s demonstrating the feasibility of changing the dyskinetic symptoms by manipulating the neurotransmitter activities at the synaptic levels. The author, along with Kazamatsuri and Cole,[7-10] in this regard, has reported on the efficacy of such agents as dopamine-depleting (tetrabenazine), dopamine-blocking (Haloperidol, Thiopropazate), dopamine-competing (alpha-methyldopa), cholinergic (Deanol), and GABA potentiating (Sodium Valproate). The findings generally supported the synaptic theory insofar that such a manipulation of transmitters could indeed bring a change in the clinical picture. Friedhoff and Alpert advocated deliberate receptor sensitivity modification (RSM) in the treatment of tardive dyskinesia, schizophrenia, and Gilles de la Tourette syndrome, all of which are assumed to have hypersensitized or hyperactive dopamine receptors. To that effect, they administered L-Dopa to these patients, with the anticipation of initial worsening followed by an eventual improvement due to the adaptive decrease in receptor sensitivity. They have found some support in their theory from the clinical results.[11] In the next decade, more information is anticipated regarding various neurotransmitters, their receptors, and the mode of action of various psychotropic drugs interacting with these transmitters and receptors at synaptic levels and the resulting neurobehavioral changes.

Neurochemistry and Neurotransmitters

The most well known studies in this area are those of depression. The catecholamine theory of depression came from two clinical observations: (1) iproniazid, originally introduced as an antiturberculosis agent, produced central nervous system stimulation and euphoria among the tubercular patients. It was found later that iproniazid was a potent inhibitor of monoamine oxidase, an enzyme largely responsible for the intraneuronal oxidation of amines in the nervous system; (2) reserpine, used as an antipsychotic and antihypertensive agent, was noticed to produce depression indistinguishable from the spontaneously occurring depression. The discovery that reserpine depleted stores of serotonin and norepinephrine in the central nervous system led to the hypothesis that biological amines in the brain play an important mood-regulating role. Several monoamine oxidase inhibitors (MAOI) have been introduced since iproniazid for the clinical management of depression. The contribution of MAOI appeared to be more to the theoretical formulation of therapeutic mechanism than to the actual clinical outcome. When norepineph-rine is released from the storage granule near the terminal of a neuron, it is destroyed by the enzyme monoamine oxidase. Large portions of norepineph-rine and other amines which are released from the nerve ending are reuptaken by the natural pumping mechanism and destroyed by the intraneuronal monoamine oxidase. Thus, inhibitors of monoamine oxidase will increase the amount of active norepinephrine available reaching the postsynaptic recep-tors. The clinical efficacy observed with tricyclic antidepressants further rein-forced the amine theory of depression. Imipramine and Amitriptyline, two prototypes of tricyclic antidepressants, were found to inhibit the reuptake of norepinphrine at the nerve ending, thus making an increased amount of physiologically active norepinephrine available to cross the synaptic cleft and reach the postsynaptic receptors. Detailed pharmacological studies revealed that desmethylimipramine, the therapeutic metabolite of imipramine, poten-tiates more norepinephrine while amitriptyline potentiates more serotonin. Such basic pharmacological properties coincide nicely with the clinical obser-vations that imipramine works more effectively for the patient with low uri-nary MHPG (3-methoxy-4-hydroxy-phenylethylene-glycol), an end metabo-lite of CNS norepinephrine, while amitriptyline works more effectively for high MHPG patients.[12] The clinical findings, that imipramine works better for retarded patients while amitriptyline works better for agitated patients, suggest that agitation may be associated with low serotonin and high norepi-nephrine levels. Psychomotor retardation could then be explained by the insufficiency of norepinephrine.

The discovery of urinary MHPG as the major parameter of norepineph-rine activities in CNS further facilitated the biochemical studies of affective disorders including mania. It was suggested that, on the basis of urinary MHPG, a subgroup of homogeneous affective disorders could be identified and treated rationally with the appropriate pharmacological agents.[13]

The technology to measure serum prolactin not only illuminates the inhibitory role of dopamine to prolactin but also provides a practical neurohormonal measurement for the blocking potential of neuroleptics at the dopamine receptors. The increase of serum prolactin is generally correlated with neuroleptic potential. Such neurohormonal parameters are more objec-tive and sensitive than the clinically manifested extrapyramidal symptoms when the potential dopamine receptor blockade of the various neuroleptics is concerned. Incidentally, because of the prolactin elevating property of neuroleptics and because of the findings of animal studies that showed that long term neuroleptic medication was associated with a higher incidence of breast cancer, the question was raised of the carcinogenic effect of neurolep-tics. The Food and Drug Administration even seriously considered requiring drug inserts to carry a warning of the possible potential of breast cancer.

However, an epidemiological survey of mental patients, who received neuroleptics, did not reveal any evidence of a higher incidence of breast cancer. The proposal for such a warning was then dropped.

Pharmacokinetics and Therapeutic Plasma Levels

With the recent development of laboratory techniques in measuring the drugs and their metabolites in the plasma and other tissue fluids, a new hope was raised as to the feasibility of practicing an objective and rational drug therapy using the plasma levels of therapeutic agents as guidelines. Such a laboratory guided therapy is welcomed by many clinicians who have been using the trial and error method for decades in determining the optimal dosage for their patients. The earlier reports of Asberg and Kragh-Sorenson from Scandinavia dramatically demonstrated the "therapeutic window" of nortriptyline.[14, 15] They showed that depressive patients responded well when the plasma levels of nortriptyline were between 50 to 180 ng/ml. Above and below these levels, patients did not improve. When they adjusted the oral dosage to bring the plasma level within the therapeutic range, the patients' clinical condition improved. They recommended, therefore, to use the plasma level as a quick guideline after only a few days of medication, rather than to wait weeks to reach optimal dosage by trial and error. Since these reports, there has been a burgeoning of plasma level studies aiming at establishing therapeutic range. The results so far are inconclusive; with the exception of nortriptyline (therapeutic range, 50 to 180 ng/ml) and probably imipramine (therapeutic plasma level, including the therapeutic metabolite, desipramine, is above 150 ng/ml without an upper limit), other psychotropic drugs were studied in small numbers of patients, or showed different levels of therapeutic range. Some studies showed no correlation at all between the plasma levels and clinical outcome. Even in lithium, the least complicated agent, i.e., without any metabolite, and relatively standardized in its laboratory procedure, the therapeutic level for mania in the United States was shown to be above 0.9 mEq/liter, while 70 percent of the Japanese mania responded well at level below 0.86 mEq/liter. The workshop on transcultural psychopharmacology held in the 1978 American College of Neuropsychopharmacology meeting raised some doubt about the applicability of therapeutic plasma levels, established for Caucasian patients, to Japanese patients.[16] The oriental patients used smaller dosages of lithium, antidepressants, and neuroleptics; and the plasma levels of these drugs were correspondingly lower than those reported in the United States, for which the majority of the data came from the Caucasian population.

Clinical outcome for the Oriental patients was reported to be quite satisfactory. Obviously more intra- and intercultural studies are needed with standardized diagnostic criteria and measurements.

The neuroleptic plasma level studies are still in their infancy and are rather disappointing so far. In contrast, the studies on tricyclic antidepressants are relatively active, probably due to the initial encouraging reports on nortriptyline from Scandinavian investigators, coupled with the fact that at best only 70 percent of the depressive patients responded to tricyclic antidepressants. Thus, studies of plasma levels provide incentive to deal with these treatment-refractory patients. With neuroleptics the situation is somewhat different. The variation of therapeutic oral dosage of neuroleptics is quite great and there are not enough identical results or confirmations as to their therapeutic plasma levels. There are still many unknown metabolites and inadequate knowledge on the metabolism of a given neuroleptic. Without clear understanding of the therapeutic role these metabolites play, merely trying to correlate the plasma levels of the parent drug to the clinical status may result in a futile, if not misleading, effort. In view of the complexities of assay and of drug metabolism, May and Van Putten advocate the test dose concept. Instead of dealing with "steady state" plasma levels, they attempted to measure the response to a single test dose. It seemed to them wise, in the first instance, to focus clinically well designed studies on the parent substance, rather than launch into more costly, but clinically unsophisticated, studies of its metabolites.[17] The attempt to shift attention from the sustained plasma levels to a single test as a way to predict the possible clinical outcome is refreshing. However, this may be applicable for a new patient prior to medication, and cannot provide laboratory guidance for the patients who have already been on maintenance medication. More data are needed to confirm the usefulness of the test dose concept.

Pharmacokinetic studies provided new information not only on the metabolites of a parent drug but also on the half-life of the drug, which could help the clinician to determine the timing of medication more rationally. The most relevant clinically pharmacokinetic studies came from antianxiety agents, particularly the benzodiazepine family. To give a few examples, intramuscular injection of diazepam was found, contrary to common belief, to be slower than oral administration in terms of plasma level elevation. This finding has contributed a great deal to the clinician's dealing with emergency management. Other factors, such as advanced age, liver cirrhosis, and sex, have been demonstrated to prolong the half-life of diazepam. This information again helps the clinician to become more sophisticated in using diazepam with various patients. In view of the wide usage of diazepam in nursing homes and for alcoholics with possible liver damage, prolonged half-life could sometimes lead to a serious accumulation of the drug in the body and elevation of plasma level to a toxic degree. Even acknowledging the relative safety and extremely high lethal dosage of diazepam, its side effects, such as ataxia and muscle weakness, could cause serious accidents to the elderly patients. Smoking and barbiturates were found to shorten the half-life of several psychotropic drugs because of the faster metabolic breakdown in the liver because of increased hepatosomal enzyme activity. These patients may require higher dosage and more frequent medication to attain the therapeutic effect. Without the contribution from pharmacokinetic studies, clinicians would still have remained with the trial and error method of treatment.

Frequency of Medication and Economy of Prescription

Psychotropic drugs, without exception, used to be administered three or four times a day in the traditional manner as with other medicinal agents. With the help of pharmacokinetic information, it is now known that the half-life of most of the psychotropic drugs is longer than that of other drugs; therefore, t.i.d or q.i.d administration is not warranted. Several clinical studies demonstrated that when t.i.d or q.i.d schedules were changed to b.i.d. or q.d., the clinical efficacy remained the same or even improved in some ways. It was also found that when two-thirds of the daily dosage was administered at bedtime, the autonomic nervous system side effects became less and the psychomotor function improved. DiMascio made a detailed cost analysis on the size of tablet and demonstrated that if a larger dose tablet were used instead of a smaller one the saving on the drug cost could be worthwhile.[18] For instance, the cost of administering 400 mg of thioridazine in different strength tablets can vary from 54.4¢ per day (four 25 mg tablets q.i.d.) to 14.5¢ per day (one 200 mg tablet b.i.d.), almost a 400 percent difference in cost. In the era of high medical cost, such information could help the physician to reduce the cost of expensive medical care.

Length of Medication

Since some schools of psychiatry view the effects of psychotropic drugs as symptom-relief, it is understandable that in the early era of psychopharmacology, medication was given only for a short period until the patient's symptoms subsided. Clinically this was satisfactory in most cases of anxiety neurosis or depression. For schizophrenia, due to its often prolonged or recurring course, continuous medication for months and years became the clinical reality. Numerous studies have been carried out to experimentally test whether such a maintenance medication is necessary. In the case of antipsychotic drugs for schizophrenia, it was found quite consistently, in most of the studies, that patients' relapse rates ranged from 40 percent to 60 percent at the end of six months and 60 percent to 80 percent at the end of one year, if they were kept without antipsychotic medication. The need of maintenance medication was thus established. In view of the possible induction of tardive dyskinesia and other undesirable side effects which are often associated with long term usage of antipsychotic drugs, the question was raised as to how long and in what manner the maintenance medication should be carried out in order to minimize the possible physical and mental risks. Although there is no literature clearly demonstrating the maximum period required for maintenance medication, many empirical reports and some controlled studies indicate that drug holiday or intermittent drug therapy could be administered quite successfully. The author has also reported the feasibility of patient self-regulated intermittent drug therapy in the landlord-supervised cooperative apartments program.[19] Psychosocial therapy was also found to have some delayed alleviating effect in the prevention of relapse when both drug and psychosocial therapy were given together.

In the well publicized NIMH collaborative outpatient study of schizophrenia, Hogarty, Goldberg and Schooler found that psychosocial treatment alone neither prevented relapse to any extent nor improved the social adjustment. They concluded that the optimum benefits, both in preventing relapse and in enhancing adjustment, require that both drug and nondrug treatments be given for more than one year.[20] Obviously, more studies are needed for the search of more effective nondrug treatment modalities so that these effect-proven nondrug therapies could supplement, or even replace, the possible life-long maintenance medication. In the area of affective disorder, long-term studies on the therapeutic and preventive effects of imipramine, lithium, and imipramine combined with lithium, for unipolar and bipolar affective disorders, are still going on. The final data will be available in the near future. Cognitive therapy, with or without antidepressants for nonpsychotic depressive patients will be tested under the auspices of NIMH.[21]

Polypharmacy

In the late 1950s and early 1960s, and even until recently, cocktail polypharmacy, mixing various antipsychotics, antidepressants and antianxiety agents, was not an unusual clinical practice. This practice was conceived because of the polymorphous nature of target symptoms and also because of the belief that a little bit of each drug in the cocktail form might reduce their respective side effects. However, the studies comparing the efficacy of single versus combined drug treatment revealed that in general, combination of different types of drugs did not appear to be more beneficial than a single drug regimen.[22,23] Except in schizoaffective or agitated affective disorders, for which the combination of antipsychotic and antidepressant drugs may be useful, almost all other psychiatric conditions requiring medication can be managed satisfactorily with one well selected drug at the right dosage. Although polypharmacy, which combines different psychotropic drugs, has been reduced in many psychiatric facilities, the combination of psychotropic drugs and other nonpsychotropic drugs in the nursing homes still presents a potential hazard. Several drug survey studies consistently pointed out that in nursing homes four or more drugs, psychiatric or nonpsychiatric, were commonly administered simultaneously to the same patient. While some of these drugs might be life-saving, the potential hazard of drug interaction, short-term or long-term, should not be neglected. Physicians should give a careful consideration of the possible risk against the benefit when they have to prescribe several drugs to a patient. Such knowledge of drug interaction can be widened if more research is carried out, particularly in the geriatric field.

Prophylactic Use of Antiparkinsonian Agents

The epidemic use of prophylactic parkinsonian agents in the United States, as seen in the 1960s, came from the assumptions that (1) extrapyramidal side effects were untherapeutic and inhumane and (2) combination of antiparkinsonian and antipsychotic drugs could prevent the manifestation of extrapyramidal symptoms. The first assumption was supported by the NIMH study in which Cole and Clyde could not find any difference in the clinical outcome when they compared thioridazine and fluphenazine in the treatment of chronic schizophrenics. Thioridazine caused extrapyramidal symptoms in 3 percent of the patients, compared with 36 percent by fluphenazine.[24] Other studies from Anglo-American schools also failed to support any positive relation between the extrapyramidal symptoms and therapeutic effect. These were important studies because they disputed the European view that manifestation of extrapyramidal symptoms was a sine qua non for the effective drug treatment of schizophrenia.

A series of controlled studies on the second assumption, as mentioned above, did not show significant effects of antiparkinsonian drugs in the prevention of extrapyramidal symptoms (EPS). Although the intensity of EPS appeared to be somewhat milder among those who took antiparkinsonian agents prophylactically than those who were not on them, the frequency of EPS seemed to be the same in both groups. Furthermore, when antiparkinsonian agents were withdrawn from the patients who had been on both neuroleptics and antiparkinsonian agents, the relapse rate of EPS was almost negligible, particularly among those who had been on such a drug regimen for longer than three months. These research findings were put into clinical practice in the Massachusetts State Hospital system. Subsequently the use of antiparkinsonian agents has been reduced from 3,500,000 tablets in 1968 to less than 1,500,000 in 1973, a reduction of 2,000,000 tablets and a saving of over $20,000 in one year. Recently drug-induced akinesia has been connected to depression.[25,26] Continuous usage of antiparkinsonian agents is justifiable for these special patients if the dosage of neuroleptic drug can not be reduced further for clinical reason.

Personality and Dynamic Concepts in Drug Response

It is commonly observed that when a physician administers a standard psychotropic drug in a standard dosage to a group of patients for whom he believes this drug to be indicated, the clinical responses of these patients often vary and rarely show identical pictures. This is understandable from the viewpoint that the overall end result of a psychotropic drug on human behavior is determined by the total interaction of pharmacology, physiology, chemistry, and the patient's own response to these drug-induced physical changes. The latter is determined by personality variables of patient and doctors, milieu, attitudes and expectation toward drugs, etc. Over the last two decades, there has emerged a growing body of literature concerning these variables. The so-called "nonspecific factors", as determinants of behavioral response to drugs, are now gaining acceptance among clinicians. Such an insight is often helpful to understand the patient's behavior during drug treatment. For example, Sarwer-Foner introduced the term "psychodynamically determined paradoxical behavioral reaction" to describe those instances in which symptoms such as panic, paranoid reaction, body image distortion, and markedly enhanced anxiety, result from drug administration. He hypothesized that ". . . the pharmacological drug effect chemically removes or interferes with activities that are used by the patient as components of major ego defenses against underlying unconscious conflicts." He further stated, "Examples of this are increased anxiety due to the passivity and immobility imposed by the drugs or alteration of bodily feelings leading to disorganization and loss of control."[27,28] Independent experimental support for this view came from studies of Heninger, DiMascio and Klerman in which a highly select group of extroverted, physically oriented athletes reacted negatively to the motor-inhibiting effects of chlorpromazine, while introverted, passive, nonphysically oriented individuals showed positive response.[29] In the United States, where dynamic psychiatry is the main stream of psychiatric thought, such information from research can be readily translated into practice.

Drugs and Psychotherapy

Since psychotherapy of various kinds and intensities has often been applied together with drug therapy, either to inpatients or outpatients, comparisons of the relative efficacy of drug therapy and of psychotherapy have received a great amount of attention in the last two decades. The negative results from two well known controlled studies, one by Grinspoon, Ewalt and Shader[30] and the other by May,[31] have led to current doubts as to the usefulness of individual psychotherapy as a treatment for schizophrenic patients. The impact and influence of these studies can be dramatically illustrated by the conflicting ethical standards held toward individual psychotherapy before and after the completion of these studies: in 1960 when the studies were being initiated, it was regarded as unethical not to give a control group psychotherapy, but by 1968 it was considered unethical to give a control group psychotherapy alone.[32] Although there were some critical comments as to the methodology of these studies, the impact on the mode of mental health delivery in the United States, if not in the world, has been significant. Currently there is another collaborative study under way in Boston that addresses many questions raised by previous research on inpatients treated by intensive psychotherapy.[32]

In the field of depression there has been, in this decade, some clear evidence as to the relative roles of psychotherapy and pharmacotherapy. Therapy, whether group, individual, or marital, was applied to ambulatory neurotic depressive patients in conjunction with tricyclic antidepressants; it was then found that whereas drug therapy was effective in preventing relapse and reducing symptoms, it had minimal or no effect on social and interpersonal functioning. On the other hand, psychotherapy was found to improve overall social functioning, empathetic understanding, and to reduce interpersonal sensitivity, but had no effect on relapse rate or symptoms.[33] Thus the two treatment modalities are supportive of each other rather than exclusive. Due to the different contribution each treatment modality provides, the combination of drugs and psychotherapy for ambulatory depressed outpatients promises to be the most efficacious treatment, providing maximum benefit. Preliminary evidence comparing drugs to cognitive therapy suggests that cognitive therapy may have some advantage over drugs in the treatment of nonpsychotic depressive patients, but it is possible that the combination could be more effective than either treatment alone. NIMH is currently planning a large scale, long term collaborative study comparing the relative efficacy of cognitive therapy to another type of psychotherapy, with or without tricyclic antidepressants in either type of psychotherapy.[21] It is hoped that in the next decade, research will bring increasingly useful answers to questions like these.

REFERENCES

1. Pharmacotherapy and Psychotherapy: Paradoxes, Problems and Progress. Formulated by the Committee on Research, Group for the Advancement of Psychiatry, Vol IX, Report No. 83, March 1975, pp. 19−20

2. Snyder SH: The dopamine hypothesis of schizophrenia: Focus on the dopamine receptor. Am. J. Psychiatry 133:197−202, 1976

3. Feinberg AP, Snyder SH: Phenothiazine drugs: Structure-activity relationships explained by a conformation that mimics dopamine. Proc. Natl. Acad. Sci., U.S.A. 72:1899−1903, 1975

4. Snyder SH, Banerjee SP, Yamamura HI, et al: Drugs, Neurotransmitters and schizophrenia. Science 184:1234−1253, 1974

5. Engel J: Pre-synaptic receptors: Basic and clinical aspects. Presented at American College of Neuropsychopharmacology, Maui, Hawaii, 1978

6. Cannon WB, and Rosenbleuth A. (eds): The Supersensitivity of Denervated Structures. MacMillan, New York, 1949, pp 1−245

7. Kazamatsuri H, Chien CP, and Cole JO: Treatment of tardive dyskinesia (I): Clinical efficacy of a dopamine-depleting agent, haloperidol and thiopropazate. Arch. Gen. Psychiatry 27 (Jul): 95−99, 1972

8. Kazamatsuri H, Chien CP, and Cole JO: Treatment of tardive dyskinesia (II): Short-term efficacy of dopamine-blocking agents, haloperidol and thiopropazate. Arch. Gen. Psychiatry 27 (Jul): 100−103, 1972

9. Kazamatsuri H, Chien CP, and Cole JO: Treatment of tardive dyskinesia (III): Clinical efficacy of a dopamine-competing agent, methyldopa. Arch. Gen. Psychiatry 27:824−827, 1972

10. Chien CP, Jung K, and Ross-Townsend A: Efficacies of agents related to GABA, dopamine and acetylcholine in tardive dyskinesia. Psychopharmacology Bulletin 14, 1978

11. Friedhoff AJ, Alpert M: Receptor sensitivity modification as a potential treatment, in Lipton MA, DiMascio A, Killam KF (eds): Psychopharmacology: A Generation of Progress. New York, Raven Press, 1978

12. Mass JW: Clinical and Biochemical Heterogeneity of Depressive Disorders. Ann. Int. Med. 88:556−563, 1978

13. Schildkraut JJ, Orsulak PJ, Schatzberg AF, Gudeman JE, Cole JO, Rohde WA, and LaBrie RA: Towards a Biochemical Classification of Depressive Disorders. Arch. Gen. Psychiatry 35:1427−1433, 1978

14. Asberg M, Cronholm B, Sjoqvist F, et al: Relationship between plasma level and therapeutic effect of nortriptyline. Br. Med. J. 3:331−334, 1971

15. Kragh-Sorenson P, Hansen CE, Baastrup PC, et al: Psychopharmacologia 45:305−312, 1976

16. Chien CP: Transcultural psychopharmacology in depression: New insights. Psychopharmacology Bulletin 15:24−45, 1979

17. May PRA, Van Putten T: Plasma levels of chlorpromazine in schizophrenia—A critical review of the literature. Arch. Gen. Psychiatry 35:1081−1087, 1978

18. DiMascio A: Innovative Drug Administration. In Ayd F (ed): Rational Psychopharmacotherapy and the Right to Treatment. Baltimore, Ayd Medical Communication, 1975 pp 118−130

19. Chien CP: Drugs and rehabilitation in schizophrenia. In Greenblatt M (ed): Drugs in Combination with Other Therapies. New York, Grune and Stratton, 1975, pp 13−34

20. Hogarty GE, Goldberg SC, Schooler NR: Drug and Sociotherapy in the After-

care of Schizophrenia: A Review. In Greenblatt M (ed): Drugs in Combination with other Therapies, Seminars in Psychiatry. New York, Grune & Stratton, 1975 pp 1–12

21. Waskow I, Hadley S, Autry J, Parloff M: Psychotherapy of Depression Collaborative Program. Division of Extramural Research Program, Clinical Research Branch, NIMH. Announcement, Dec., 1978

22. Freeman H: The therapeutic value of combinations of psychotropic drugs. A Review. Psychopharmacol. Bull. 4:1–27, 1967

23. Merlis S, et al: Polypharmacy in psychiatry: Patterns of differential treatment. Am. J. Psychiatry 126:1647–1651, 1970

24. Cole JO, Clyde DJ: Extrapyramidal side effects and clinical response to phenothiazines. Rev. Can. Biol. 20:565–574, 1961

25. Van Putten T, May PRA: Akinetic depression in schizophrenia. Arch. Gen. Psychiatry 35:1101–1107, 1978

26. Rifkin A, Quitkin F, Klein DF: Akinesia. Arch. Gen. Psychiatry 32:672–674, 1975

27. Sarwer-Foner GJ: Recognition and management of drug-induced "extrapyramidal" reaction and "paradoxical" behavioral reactions in psychiatry. Can. Med. Assoc. J. 83:312–318, 1960

28. Sarwer-Foner GJ: Some comments on the psychodynamic aspects of the extrapyramidal system and neuroleptics. Montreal, Editions Psychiatriques, 1961

29. Heninger G, DiMascio A, and Klerman G: Personality factors in variability of response to phenothiazines. Am. J. Psychiat. 121:1091–1094, 1965

30. Grinspoon L, Ewalt JR, Shader RI: Schizophrenia: Pharmacotherapy and psychotherapy. Baltimore, Williams & Wilkins, 1972

31. May PRA: Treatment of Schizophrenia. New York, Science House, 1968

32. Mosher LR, Keith SJ: Research on the psychosocial treatment of schizophrenia: A summary report. Am. J. Psychiatry 136:623–631, 1979

33. Weissman MM: Psychotherapy and its relevance to the pharmacotherapy of affective disorders: From ideology to evidence. In Lipton M, DiMascio A, Killam K (eds): Psychopharmacology—A Generation of Progress. New York, Raven Press, 1977

Lawrence F. Gosenfeld
Barbara E. Ehrlich
Jared M. Diamond

5
Affective Disorders and Lithium

Zubin, in an elegant cross cultural study comparing the United States and the United Kingdom, showed that American psychiatrists tended to label as schizophrenic what their British counterparts termed manic-depressive illness.[1] While this may once have been academic, it now becomes a matter of critical importance since it has been pointed out by numerous investigators that the response to treatment and the future prognosis of the manic-depressive patient treated with lithium can be good to excellent, contrasted to the schizophrenic whose prognosis is usually poor and whose illness normally results in deterioration and decreased social functioning. Mendelwicz has pointed out that bipolar patients with family history of mania (FH+) tend to be lithium responders, whereas bipolar patients with a negative family history of mania and depression (FH−) do not respond as readily. He has offered some differentiation that leads one to believe that criteria for defining a medical syndrome, its etiology, its course, its epidemiology and possibly its treatment, can eventually be fulfilled.[2]

HISTORY OF AFFECTIVE DISORDERS

Kraepelin, writing about manic-depressive illness, stated, "Usually all morbid manifestations completely disappear but where that is not the case, only a rather slight, peculiar psychic weakness develops, which is just as common to the types here taken together as it is different from dementias in diseases of other kinds."[3] Twenty-one years later in 1942, Rennie published a paper based on a study of 208 manic-depressive patients admitted to the Phipps Clinic from 1913 to 1916. He pointed out that 93 percent of the Phipps patients recovered from the first attack even though 79 percent had recurrences. Of these original 208, 11 or 5 percent committed suicide. Two of these were patients in manic phase with no depressive content at that time.[4] Recently, Glen published a paper on mortality of lithium treated patients and found that of 784 patients, suicide was one of the most common causes of death with 8 cases or 1 percent.[5] The expected incidence if these patients were not on lithium would be 41.5 by extrapolation. This figure is significant at the $p < .001$ level. We use this as a simple gross statistical evaluation to hint that lithium may be life saving because of its most important effect: prophylaxis of severe endogenous depression in bipolar patients, which may otherwise lead to suicide.

Prang in an article has facetiously pointed out that if one observes 100 randomly selected depressed patients per month, he will find that 25 will recover spontaneously, 25 more will recover if they are given a placebo, another 25 will recover if given an appropriate drug, and 25 will remain sick whatever is done. "The first 50 provide baseline gratification for the physician but confound research; the next 25 reward the pharmacological therapist, and the final 25 are a source of general frustration."[6] As John Davis has pointed out in the past, "We are currently in a state of parapsychopharmacology; we observe, measure and report a great deal, and know very little about what is really going on."[7] The specific etiologic considerations for most mental conditions have not been identified as yet and classification therefore rests on symptomatology and clinical course. The deficiencies of validity and reliability are increasingly obvious, especially with reference to biological research. Our focus here on current advances in research into manic-depressive illness is with particular advances in understanding the actions of lithium on the body. It ignores the question of whether lithium is disease specific or symptom specific.

At one time, numerous medical illnesses masqueraded as psychiatric symptoms and were thought to belong to the dementias. In reviewing those illnesses thought to have been psychiatric, one can count hypo- and hyperthyroidism, Cushing's syndrome, Pellagra and drug (licit and illicit) induced psychosis. The same may be true of affective disorders today in that we have depressive illness with its vast spectrum, schizoaffective schizophrenia both depressed and manic, manic-depressive type I and II, and manic-depressive lithium responsive and non-responsive. This would not be critical except that diagnosis itself is not consistent, and as a consequence neither is current treatment.

In the ancient textbooks such as Symptom Diagnosis, 5th Edition, 1961,[8] and in Harrison's Principles of Internal Medicine, 2nd Edition, Volume I,

1953,[9] each of these then-current textbooks devotes less than two pages to diagnosis and treatment of manic-depressive psychosis. Nowhere in these editions is the word lithium mentioned. Essentially, between the time of Kraepelin's description of manic-depressive illness and the resurgence of research commencing in 1965, the diagnosis of manic-depressive illness seemed to be totally dying out in the United States.

PROBLEMS OF DIAGNOSIS

In trying to define a clinical syndrome, there are recognized factors which describe the ideal picture. A definable syndrome should have (1) typical signs and symptoms, including biochemical and pathological findings; (2) onset at a recognizable time, hopefully with a characteristic course; (3) a definable outcome or prognosis; (4) knowledge of epidemiology; (5) etiology; and (6) treatment.

Excluding the debate of differential diagnostic problems between other countries and the United States, since the introduction of lithium there has been an epidemic of manic-depressive illness in this country. Whether this is a change in education and practice, or whether we are more eager to place people on lithium who might respond, there is definitely an upward trend.

Three issues emerge as prime aspects of research into this simple positive ion reported by Cade in 1949.[10] First, and of primary importance for the clinician, is diagnosis. Second, the mechanism of action (the greatest hope of understanding etiology of a subgroup of psychiatric disorders), and third, long term side effects and toxicity of this remarkably simple medication. These issues will probably remain unsolved for the ensuing ten years.

Of the approximately 60 patients currently on lithium therapy in the Affective Disorders Clinic at the Brentwood Veterans Administration Medical Center, only two carried the initial diagnosis of manic-depressive illness. This is an unremarkable 3 percent of the population in this clinic. If patients would present like childrens' building blocks, i.e., either purely circular or purely square, the issue would have been resolved. Unfortunately, there are schizophrenics who display affective symptoms and, more importantly, manic patients who present schizophreniform symptoms. The problem has been most recently brought into focus by Edelstein[11] and Garver.[12] These papers make use of two previously reported conditions observed in treating schizophrenic patients of good prognosis with affective symptoms. In the report by Edelstein, patients were given injections of 4 mg physostigmine I.V. and rated on a blind basis. Fifteen minutes following physostigmine infusion, those who were rated as good prognosis schizophrenics (N = 4) and who were subsequently lithium responders showed a reduction of Brief Psychiatric Rating

Scale (BPRS) thought disorder of 46 percent ± 16 percent. In contrast, poor prognosis schizophrenics, lithium nonresponders (N = 4), showed a 17 percent ± 11 percent worsening of symptoms with p < .02 by the two-tailed t-test.

David Garver also pointed out other indicators of responsiveness in this schizophrenic-like group that we will refer to later.[12] Even with the biological classifications which research is attempting to define, the best indicators at present for response to lithium seem to be past history and features of good prognosis schizophrenia. That is, the type of individual who seems to do well on lithium is an individual with a good premorbid history or one without a premorbid history of schizophrenia, with a family history that is likely not schizophrenic, but leans more towards an affective illness, and who shows good illness interface, i.e., personality restoration when not acutely ill and no intellectual deterioration.[13,14] This would be a patient who exhibits spontaneous remission. In summary, then, when one fails to consider the course of the illness, the cognitive status, and the present functioning of the patient, the results are often misdiagnosis and, as a consequence, inappropriate pharmacological regimes.

RED BLOOD CELL LITHIUM TRANSPORT

After a diagnosis of manic depressive illness is made, lithium is the preferred treatment. Although lithium's mechanism of action is unknown, Mendels and Frazer suggested a membrane-based theory after describing higher lithium cell-to-plasma concentration ratios in bipolar depressed patients who responded than in those who did not respond.[15] Interest in intracellular lithium led to investigation of lithium transport across erythrocyte (RBC) membrane by mechanisms previously shown to carry other cations.[16-19] These mechanisms are: The Na^+—K^+ ATPase, Na^+—Li^+ countertransport, a bicarbonate-sensitive pathway, and a leak. While all can be shown to transport lithium under in vitro conditions, i.e., nonphysiological concentrations of lithium, sodium or potassium, our findings suggested that in situations that simulate in vivo conditions, influx is predominantly by the leak and efflux is predominantly by the Na^+—Li^+ countertransport (Fig. 5-1).

Fortuitously, we were able to study lithium transport in RBC from a pair of twins. This study suggested that both genetic and nongenetic (lithium-induced) factors control countertransport efflux. The lithium ratio was measured in a pair of male monozygotic twins.[20] Both were diagnosed manic-depressive disorder (RDC Criteria). When both twins were taking lithium, values for lithium ratio appeared closer in the twins (0.39± 0.05 versus 0.42;

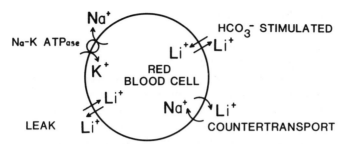

Fig. 5-1. Red blood cell lithium transport mechanisms. These four mechanisms can be shown to transport lithium under in vitro conditions. In situations that simulate in vivo conditions, however, influx is predominantly by the leak and efflux is predominantly by the Na^+—Li^+ countertransport.

mean ± SD for one twin, a single measurement for the other twin) than would be expected from random pairs of lithium treated individuals (range, 0.20 to 0.95).[21] Among individuals, variation in the rate of lithium leak is negligible, while the rate of countertransport varies nearly six-fold.[21] The closeness of the lithium ratios measured in the twins suggests that their countertransport rates are also similar and that countertransport is a genetic control of the lithium efflux rate. We then measured lithium transport in vitro in RBC samples from the twins one month after one brother had stopped lithium treatment while the other brother had been taking lithium carbonate, 2100 mg per day, continuously for 2.5 years. Efflux via the Na^+—Li^+ countertransport mechanism in the brother who was not taking lithium was comparable to maximal values measured in our laboratory for normal individuals not on lithium therapy.[22] This countertransport fraction of efflux was 19 percent lower in the lithium treated brother. A decrease of this magnitude in the lithium treated brother is significant for two reasons: (1) countertransport flux shows little variation over time when measured in vitro in RBC from the same healthy individual, and; (2) no other differences in transport parameters were detected between the RBC samples of the twins. The difference in countertransport efflux between the treated and untreated twins suggests that the presence or absence of lithium therapy affects lithium efflux rates. Our results showed that the maximum rate of lithium efflux depends on at least two factors: (1) the maximum rate of Na^+—Li^+ countertransport, which may be under genetic control, and; (2) the presence or absence of lithium treatment. The degree of lithium-induced decrease in Na^+—Li^+ countertransport varies among individuals and can be as large as 50 percent. Other studies have confirmed these findings.[24,25]

CHOLINE TRANSPORT IN THE RBC

Results of this sort led us to examine other transport deficiencies relative to affective disorders. For example, an irreversible decrease in the transport of choline has been reported.[26] This compound is important as a precursor for acetylcholine and the membrane phospholipid phosphatidylcholine.

In trying to determine why the influx of choline was so drastically reduced, we measured the endogenous levels of choline in plasma and RBC. The results obtained were very unexpected.[27] Plasma choline concentrations for both normal subjects and lithium-treated patients were comparable, averaging $15\mu M$. However, the RBC choline concentration in 7 untreated subjects averaged $50 \pm 4\mu M$, while the 5 lithium-treated subjects had levels of $420 \pm 10\mu M$. This is a ten-fold increase in intracellular choline concentration, with no change in plasma choline concentration and no overlap of the cell values between treated and untreated subjects. The time course of the change in intracellular choline was studied in a manic-depressive patient initially drug-free. On admission, plasma and RBC choline concentrations were 12.4 and $52.8\mu M$, respectively. While plasma concentration stayed constant, RBC choline increased to 160, 296, 345 μM after one, two, and three weeks of lithium therapy, respectively. Lithium in plasma and RBC were relatively constant after the first week. This patient was followed for twelve weeks with no further changes in choline or lithium concentration. Although there is no direct evidence, it is suggested that the primary defect in choline transport is a decrease in efflux similar to that measured in Na^+—Li^+ countertransport after initiation of lithium therapy.

CHOLINE TRANSPORT IN THE BRAIN

To see if the decreased choline transport measure in RBC was unique to RBC, we then looked at choline transport in blood−brain barrier and synaptosomes. The major role of the blood−brain barrier is to control the composition of the cerebrospinal fluid. Normally, the blood−brain barrier regulates ions, nutrients, and metabolites in cerebrospinal fluid within narrow limits, because the cerebrospinal fluid is in direct contact with central nervous system neurons. Alterations in the composition of this extracellular fluid may affect synaptic events or may change neurofunction.

We used two techniques to try to quantitate the changes of choline in the blood−brain barrier. We used the technique of Oldendorf to calculate the brain uptake index (BUI) of choline, tyrosine, and tryptophan in rats treated for two weeks with lithium when compared with control rats.[28] The lithium treated rats had a 20 percent decrease in the BUI for choline (the brain uptake index is in effect the measurement of the uptake of a substance across the blood−brain barrier relative to the uptake of water which passes readily). The BUI for tyrosine and tryptophan were not changed. The second technique examined steady state choline accumulation in frog arachnoid and choroid plexus. We found that lithium did not alter the choline accumulation in choroid plexus; however, it greatly reduced uptake in the arachnoid.[29] This was not altogether surprising since the arachnoid is the major route of efflux from the brain while the choroid plexus does not play an important role in choline metabolism.[30] These experiments suggest a reduced turnover of choline in the brain which may elevate the choline level intracellularly similar to that seen in the RBC.

Choline is important as a precursor of acetylcholine production. Jope examined the high affinity uptake in synaptosomes of lithium treated rats. He concluded that both higher affinity uptake and ACh production were increased in lithium treated rats.[31]

These series of experiments imply that lithium may be changing the membrane transport process that controls ionic composition and may therefore alter neurotransmitter concentrations in the brain. These results are mirrored in the RBC which, while probably not directly related to affective disorder, is the most readily accessible cell which may be safely and repeatedly sampled.

The accumulation of choline noted in the foregoing experiments contributes additional information regarding the effect of lithium on the treatment and possible prophylaxis of manic-depressive disorders. If a fit is attempted to the three current theories of affective illness, i.e., catecholamine, indolamine, and cholinergic adrenergic, the latter best fits our results. Schildkraut has currently reviewed his catecholamine hypothesis,[32] and Murphy has reviewed the current status of the indolamine hypothesis of these brain neurotransmitters.[33] The entire spectrum of these neurotransmitters accounts for only 12 percent to 15 percent of neurotransmission, although in specific areas such as the corpus striatum, 15 percent of synapses are estimated to be dopaminergic.[34] The classic paper by Davis and Janowsky seems best to account for the plethora of data seen in affective disorders in humans and the animal models tested.[35] The evidence of changes in ACh metabolism and its effect on behavior and mood require mention although the hypothesis is far from proven. Schildkraut has pointed out that an all encompassing theory is not required nor should it be proposed until more evidence is available.[32] The concept of ACh relative excess accounting for depression or an adrenergic deficiency relative to ACh balance is not inconsistent with other theories and does account for other observations. Likewise the calming seen when ACh levels are raised with physostigmine in hyperactive humans whether endogenously induced (manic) or chemically induced (amphetamines) does aid in understanding the current available evidence of chemically mediated human behavior.

The effects of lithium on brain neurotransmitters in all the systems mentioned are well outlined in Neuroscience Bulletin.[36] Effects are noted for norepinephrine, acetylcholine, and serotonin. While none of the theories accounts for the vast possibilities, they all allow room for conceptualization. Factors such as alteration of membrane permeability, postsynaptic sensitivity, and enzyme system changes can easily be incorporated.

PHARMACOKINETIC MODEL OF DISTRIBUTION

In our latest experiments we have improved the pharmacokinetic model of lithium's distribution in the body. In our model, the body is divided into extracellular fluid and two different cell types rather than a single cell type represented by RBC. In performing single dose experiments, we measured changes in lithium concentration in plasma, RBC, and urine. In this way more compartments could be monitored simultaneously than in previous studies.[37] The compartmental approach of lithium pharmacokinetics was extended so that the generated parameters of distribution could be related to physiological transport processes (Fig. 5-2). From the generated parameters it can be determined where lithium has accumulated and how different cells handle lithium as a function of time. This, hopefully, can be used as a parameter for predicting optimal patient dose regimes.[38] In optimizing dose regimens several criteria can be taken into account. For example, the number of doses taken per day can be minimized to aid in patient compliance, while also trying to narrow the peak plasma level after ingestion to reduce possible side effects which may be related to large fluctuations in plasma lithium concentration (one possible side effect of this nature is long term renal pathology).[39] As a demonstration

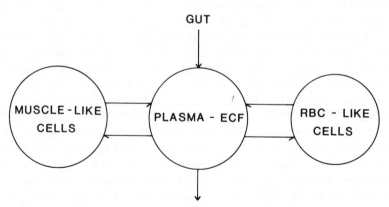

Fig. 5-2. Lithium pharmacokinetic model.

of the way pharmacokinetic parameters can be used we offer one example: since the lithium clearance varies in a diurnal fashion,[37,40] patients will maintain a peak plasma level longer if the total dose is given at night than if the maximal dose were given in the morning when clearance was higher.

KIDNEY PATHOLOGY

Pharmacokinetic analysis certainly would have practical implications vis à vis the wide-ranging controversy regarding kidney pathology reported by some investigators, most notably Hestbech, et al.[40] and could affect treatment practices. The noted lesions of focal cortical fibrosis were not correlated with age or length of treatment. The lesions noted were not specific and are of the type found in various forms of chronic nephropathy. All studied patients (147 male, 7 female) had various complications, i.e., acute intoxication or polyuria. They state, "It is possible that chronic renal disease may only develop in patients in whom the renal concentrations of lithium periodically or continually reach toxic values."[41] We studied a pair of monozygotic twins both diagnosed (RDC) manic-depressive and on lithium. One twin became toxic with serum lithium rising to 4.0 mEq/liter The second twin's lithium level remained within normal range. Biopsy of the first twin did indicate interstitial fibrosis with impaired renal functioning, creatinine clearance one-third of expected normal, nine months after lithium was discontinued. The second twin's biopsy also showed interstitial fibrosis but he never developed toxic serum levels and serum creatinine clearance was close to normal values.[42] We interpret this to mean that unless serum lithium rises to abnormally high values, chronic lithium use will not necessarily cause permanent renal damage.

PREDICTIVE BLOOD TESTS

A recent paper by Ramsey[43] brings us back to the original philosopher's stone in psychiatry, i.e., a simple in vitro test of easily accessible body fluids (like blood) to confirm a diagnosis and indicate quantity and quality of treatment. Empirical observations that manic patients tend to require higher doses of lithium to achieve therapeutic serum levels and that patients fully in remission (euthymia) could achieve similar serum levels with diminished doses of lithium led many groups to explore the relationship of intracellular lithium as measured in the RBC to that of plasma (lithium ratio). As we have pointed out earlier, the accumulation of lithium in the RBC is probably genetically determined and can be modified by treatment with lithium itself. The ratio appears to be relatively stable for each individual. Blacks and females also seem to show higher ratios.[15]

Ramsey points out the difficulty of predicting the future course of many unipolar depressives who are later found to be bipolar manic-depressives.[43] Grouped together, the differences pointed out may account for the continued controversy regarding the clinical significance of the lithium ratio.

In Mendel's original paper published in 1973[44] drawing from Serry and others' previous work[45], the concept was proposed that the lithium ratio might be predictive of lithium responsiveness in depressed patients. Lyttkens reported similar high ratios in manic patients with the highest occurring in manic females.[46] Rybakowski was not able to confirm his finding.[47] Others, including ourselves, have attempted to confirm this finding but as yet, there is no consensus.[15,48–56] We would have to agree, however, with one statement made by Ramsey, "In our experience, low-ratio bipolar patients are uncommon."[43]

NEW RESEARCH CONSIDERATIONS

What factors might account for the apparent disparity found by many workers in this field? First, the actual measurement of intracellular lithium itself is highly variable. Several groups who report negative results use indirect measurement for intracellular lithium.[49,52,55] Ehrlich and Diamond reported a method which increased the sensitivity of measurement to 10^{-13} moles with a coefficient of variation of 4 percent.[57] This improvement of five orders of magnitude over previous techniques allows numerous replicate measurements on small samples of blood. Other indirect techniques may produce errors of measurement ranging from 9 percent to 50 percent, with the greatest errors occurring at the lowest intracellular concentrations (such as found in the early stages of treatment).

Some authors have accepted lithium levels ranging as low as 0.5 mEq/liter plasma based on the assumption that the cell-to-plasma ratio is linear at all concentrations of lithium. Most of the earlier papers do not report the time between last dose and time of collection. Clinical states (depressed, manic, euthymic) are not accounted for. The problems of diagnosis are not always accounted for, although in recent papers the Research and Diagnostic Criteria (RDC) of Spitzer and Endicott[58] have become more prevalent. Even using these criteria, the premorbid adjustment is not accounted for, a factor mentioned by Garver,[12] unless the SADS-L is also used.[59]

Further factors may be of more importance, such as the new interest in choline concentrations of the red blood cell and its relation to mania. There are reports by ourselves and others of a higher than normal concentration of red cell choline in untreated manics and a marked increase of red cell choline in lithium-treated manics.[29]

RESEARCH DIAGNOSIS

RDC (Table 5−1) is an attempt to classify major psychiatric illness in a systematic way which will allow for data collected at one center to be compared to that of another. The criteria are somewhat exclusive in that they eliminate numerous patients who also display soft signs of schizophrenia, but they do develop a particular discrete population for comparison from other centers.

A further development along these lines, also by the same group, is the Schedule of Affective Disorders and Schizophrenia (SADS-L), which is a comprehensive life history of the patient.[59] While this does not modify the above RDC diagnosis it is a useful (although time consuming) longitudinal history of the patient which may also point to factors which can hopefully help differentiate between good prognosis schizophrenia (possibly an atypical or less rigorously defined affective illness) and those premorbid factors which characterize schizophrenia.

A hypothetical clinical analogy may serve to illustrate the problem. Let us assume that 100, 70 kg., 30-year-old white males, all born in Los Angeles, are admitted for treatment of fever of unknown origin (FUO) with a new experimental drug. According to Prang, 25 recover spontaneously, 25 recover on placebo, 25 recover on the new drug, and 25 stay the same or die.[7] Unless an astute observer notes that the 25 who respond to the new drug were all at one time or another in the Canal Zone in 1910 or thereabouts, the new drug Quinine is proven to be useless and aspirin will be more efficacious. Thus, until the common denominator of lithium responsive affective illness is discovered, the question may never be settled. One approach we will probably examine when sufficient data are gathered is, what do the high ratio responders to lithium have in common? As outlined, there are clearly too many differences to examine at present. Another approach would be a large collaborative study, using reproducible and standardized criteria with one facility possibly measuring lithium ratios. Patients should have a good premorbid history, a picture of social functioning at an acceptable level between episodes, a positive family history for affective illness, and the ability to remain well over a year's time while on lithium at a serum level greater than 0.9 mEq/liter. (This arbitrary figure assumes a Standard Deviation of ±0.2 mEq/liter at the laboratory measuring the clinical samples of plasma used to guide the psychiatrist in therapy, i.e., an actual range of 0.7 to 1.1 mEq/liter.) The cost of such a project will be large, but the promise of a

Table 5-1
Research and Diagnostic Criteria—Manic Disorder
(May immediately precede or follow Major Depressive Disorder.)

This category is for an episode of illness characterized by predominantly elevated, expansive, or irritable mood accompanied by the manic syndrome. It should also be used for mixed states in which manic and depressive features occur together, or when a subject cycles from a period of major depressive disorder to a period of manic disorder, or the reverse, in which case the duration recorded here should refer to the manic symptoms only. The duration of the major depressive disorder would be recorded later. Also the duration of the entire affective episode and the type of cycling is recorded later.

A through E are required for the episode of illness being considered.

A. One or more distinct periods with a predominantly elevated, expansive, or irritable mood. The elevated, expansive, or irritable mood must be a prominent part of the illness and relatively persistent although it may alternate with depressive mood. Do not include if apparently due to alcohol or drug use.

B. If mood is elevated or expansive, at least three of the following symptom categories must be definitely present to a significant degree, four if mood is only irritable. (For past episodes, because of memory difficulty, one less symptom is required.) Do not include if apparently due to alcohol or drug use.
   (1) More active than usual—either socially, at work, at home, sexually, or physically restless
   (2) More talkative than usual or felt a pressure to keep talking
   (3) Flight of ideas (as defined in this manual) or subjective experience that thoughts are racing
   (4) Inflated self-esteem (grandiosity, which may be delusional)
   (5) Decreased need for sleep
   (6) Distractibility, i.e., attention is too easily drawn to unimportant or irrelevant external stimuli
   (7) Excessive involvement in activities without recognizing the high potential for painful consequences, e.g., buying sprees, sexual indiscretions, foolish business investments, reckless driving.

C. Overall disturbance is so severe that at least one of the following is present:
   (1) Meaningful conversation is impossible
   (2) Serious impairment socially, with family, at home, at school, or at work
   (3) In the absence of (1) or (2), hospitalization.

D. Duration of manic features at least one week beginning with the first noticeable change in the subject's usual condition.

E. None of the following which suggest Schizophrenia is present. (Do not include if apparently due to alcohol or drug use.)
   (1) Delusions of being controlled (or influenced), or thought broadcasting, insertion, or withdrawal (as defined in this manual).

Table 5—1 continued.

(2) Non-affective hallucinations of any type (as defined in this manual) throughout the day for several days or intermittently throughout a one week period.

(3) Auditory hallucinations in which either a voice keeps up a running commentary on the subject's behaviors or thoughts as they occur, or two or more voices converse with each other.

(4) At some time during the period of illness had more than one week when he exhibited no prominent manic symptoms but had several instances of marked formal thought disorder (as defined in this manual), accompanied by either blunted or inappropriate affect, delusions or hallucinations of any type, or grossly disorganized behavior.

Reprinted with permission. From Spitzer RL, Endicott J, Robins E: Research Diagnostic Criteria (RDC) for a Selected Group of Functional Disorders. NIMH Clinical Research Branch. pp 14—15.

definitive biological test for a particular illness or group of illnesses cannot be discounted.

Cade, referring to the adverse reactions reported in issue 12, March, 1949, of the Journal of the American Medical Association, stated, "So in March 1949 lithium was effectively excommunicated as a therapeutic substance in the U.S." He went on to comment on the 20-year lag between his original report of lithium's use in mania and its acceptance by the medical community: "The claim was made by an unknown psychiatrist, with no research experience, working alone in a small chronic mental hospital using primitive techniques and negligible equipment."[60] So was born the first specific treatment for a psychiatric disorder. Will mania someday be called acetylcholine hyposecretion deficiency? Whatever the answer, the story of lithium is not yet over.

REFERENCES

1. Zubin J: Cross national study of diagnosis of the mental disorders: Methodology and planning. Am. J of Psychiatry (Apr. Suppl) 125:12—20, 1969

2. Mendelwicz J, Fieve RR, et al: Manic depressive illness: A comparative study of patients with and without a family history. Br. J of Psychiatry 120:523, 1972

3. Kraepelin E: Manic Depressive Insanity and Paranoia. Edinburgh, ES Livingston, 1921, p 3

4. Rennie TAC: Prognosis in manic depressive psychosis. Am J of Psychiatry 98:801, 1942

5. Glen AIM, Dodd M, Hulme EB, Kreitman N: Mortality on lithium. Neuropsychobiology 5:169—173, 1979

6. Prang AJ Jr: The use of drugs in depression: Its theoretical and practical basis. Psychiatric Annals 3:19, 1973

7. Davis JM: Personal communication, 1977–1978

8. Yater WM, WF Oliver (eds): Symptom Diagnosis (ed 5). New York, Appleton-Century-Crofts, 1961

9. Harrison TR (ed): Principles of Internal Medicine (ed 2, vol I). New York, McGraw-Hill, 1953

10. Cade CFJ: Lithium salts in the treatment of psychotic excitement. Med J Aust 36:349–352, 1949

11. Edelstein P, University of Cincinnatti College of Medicine: Physostigmine and lithium response in schizophrenia. Paper (NR25) in Proceedings of the American Psychiatric Association Conference, Chicago, 1979

12. Garver DL, University of Cincinnatti College of Medicine: The lithium ratio, lithium response. Paper (NR26) in Proceedings of the American Psychiatric Association Conference, Chicago, 1979

13. Abrams R, Taylor FA: Mania and schizoaffective disorder, manic type: A comparison. Am J of Psychiatry 133:1445–1446, 1976

14. Welner A, Croughan J, Fishman R, Robbins E: The group of schizoaffective and related psychoses: A follow-up study. Comprehensive Psychiatry 18:413–422, 1977

15. Mendels, J, Frazer A, Baron J, et al: Intraerythrocyte lithium concentration and long-term maintenance treatment. Lancet 1:966, 1976

16. Duhm J, Eisenried F, Becker BF, Griel W: Studies on the lithium transport across the red cell membrane. Pflugers Arch 364:147–155, 1976

17. Haas M, Schooler J, Tosteson DC: Coupling of lithium to sodium transport in human red cells. Nature 258:425–427, 1975

18. Pandey GN, Sarkadi B, Haas M, et al: Lithium transport pathways in human red blood cells. J Gen Physiol 72:233–247, 1978

19. Ostrow DG, Pandey GN, Davis JM, et al: A heritable disorder of lithium transport in erythrocytes of a subpopulation of manic depressive patients. Am J of Psychiatry 135:1070–1078, 1978

20. Ehrlich BE, Diamond JM, Kaye W, et al: Lithium transport in erythrocytes from a pair of twins with manic disorder. Am J of Psychiatry 136:1477–1478, 1979

21. Doris E, Pandey GN, Davis JM: Genetic determinant of lithium ion distribution: An in vitro and in vivo monozygotic-dizygotic twin study. Arch Gen Psychiatry 32:1097–1102, 1975

22. Duhm J, Becker B: Studies of the lithium transport across the red cell membrane, intra-individual variations in the Na-dependent lithium countertransport system of human erythrocytes. Pflugers Archives 370:211–219, 1977

23. Ehrlich BE, Diamond JM: Lithium fluxes in human erythrocytes. Am J of Physiology 237:C102–110, 1979

24. Ehrlich BE, Diamond JM, Clausen C, et al: The red cell membrane as a model for studying lithium's therapeutic action, in TB Cooper, S Gershon, NS Klein, M Schou (eds): Lithium: Controversies and Unresolved Issues. Amsterdam, Excerpta Medica, 1979, pp 758–767

25. Meltzer H, Rossoff CF, Kassir S, Fieve RR: Repression of the lithium pump as a

consequence of lithium ingestion by manic depressive subjects. Psychopharmacology 54:113−118, 1977

26. Lingsch C, Kaye M: An irreversible effect of lithium administration to patients. Br J of Pharmacology 57:323−327, 1976

27. Jope RS, Jenden DJ, Ehrlich BE, Diamond JM: Choline accumulates in erythrocyte during lithium therapy. N Eng J Med 299:833−834, 1978

28. Oldendorf WH: Measurement of brain uptake of radiolabeled substances using a titrated water internal standard. Brain Res 24:372−376, 1970

29. Ehrlich BE, Wright EM, Diamond JM: in preparation

30. Wright EM: Regulation of weak acids and bases in the cerebrospinal fluid. J Physiol 272:30−31, 1977

31. Jope RS, Jenden DJ: Lithium and cholenergic function in rat brain. Proceedings of the International Congress of Pharmacology, Paris, July 1978

32. Schildkraut J: Current status of the catecholamine hypothesis of affective disorders, in MA Lipton, A Di Mascio, KR Killam (eds): Psychopharmacology: A Generation of Progress. New York, Raven Press, 1948, pp 1223−1234

33. Murphy DL, Campbell F, Costa JL: Current status of the indoleamine hypothesis of the affective disorders, in MA Lipton, A Di Mascio, KRR Killam (eds): Psychopharmacology: A Generation of Progress. New York, Raven Press, 1948, pp 1235−1247

34. Suyner S: Basic science of psychopharmacology, in AM Freeman, HP Kaplan, Sadoch BJ, R Estin (eds): Comprehensive Textbook of Psychiatry, Baltimore, Williams and Wilkins, 1975, pp 104−108

35. Davis JM, Janowsky D: Cholinergic and adrenergic balance in mania and schizophrenia, in EF Domino, JM Davis (eds): Neurotransmitter Balance Regulating Behavior. Ann Arbor, EF Domino and JM Davis, 1975, pp 135−148

36. Bunney Jr. WE, Murphy DL: The Neurobiology of lithium. Neuroscience Research Program Bulletin (vol 14, #2), 165−173

37. Pauss IR, Mallinger AG, Mallinger J, Himmelhoch JM, Hanin I: Pharmacokinetics of lithium in human plasma and erythrocytes. Psychopharmacology Communications 2:91−103, 1976

38. Ehrlich BE, Clausen C, Diamond JM: Pharmacokinetics: Single dose lithium experiments, a physiological model, and improved analytical procedures. J Pharmacokinet Biopharm, in press

39. Amidsen A, Schou M: Biochemistry of depression. Lancet 1:507, 1967

40. Smith DF: Diurnal variations of lithium clearance in the rat. International Pharmacopsychiatry 8:99−103, 1973

41. Hestbech H, Hansen HE, Amidsen A, Olsen S: Chronic renal lesions following long-term treatment with lithium. Kidney International 12:205−213, 1977

42. Gosenfeld L, Ehrlich BE, Diamond JM, Kaufman-Diamond S, Dubin P: Lithium renal function, toxicity, and nocturnal enuresis. Proceedings of APA Session on Lithium Basic Mechanisms and Clinical Therapies, Atlanta, May 1978.

43. Ramsey TA, Frazer A, Mendels J, Dyson L: The erythrocyte lithium-plasma lithium ratio in patients with primary affective disorders. Arch Gen Psychiatry 36:457−461, 1975

44. Mendels J, Frazer A: Intracellular lithium concentration and clinical response.

Towards a membrane theory of depression. J of Psychiatric Research 10:9−18, 1973

45. Serry M: The lithium excretion test: Clinical application and interpretation. Aust, NZ J of Psychiatry 3:390, 1969

46. Lyttkens L, Soderberg U, Wetterberg L: Increased lithium erythrocyte/plasma ratios in manic depressive psychosis. Lancet, 1:40, 1973

47. Rybakowski J, Chtopacka M, Kupelski Z, et al: Red blood cell lithium index in patients with affective disorders in the course of lithium prophylaxis. International Pharmacopsychiatry 9:166−171, 1944

48. Albrecht VJ, Muller-Oerlinghausen B: The clinical relevance of lithium determination in the RBC: Results of a catamnestic study. Arzneim Forsch 26:1145−1147, 1976

49. Carroll BJ, Fernberg MP: Intracellular lithium. Proceedings of the American Psychiatric Association Conference, Toronto, May 5, 1977

50. Casper RC, Pandey G, Gosenfeld L, et al: Intracellular lithium and clinical response. Lancet 2:418−419, 1976

51. Demisch VL, Bochnik JH: On improved prophylaxis of endogenous-phasic psychoses: Aspects of parallel determination of lithium in serum and erythrocytes. Arzneim Forsch 26:1149−1151, 1976

52. Flemenbaum A, Weddige R, Miller J: Lithium erythrocyte/plasma ratio as a predictor of response. Am J of Psychiatry 135:336−338, 1978

53. Mendelwicz J, Verbanck P: Lithium ratio and clinical response in manic-depressive illness. Lancet 1:41, 1977

54. Rybakowski J, Strzyzewski W: Red-blood-cell lithium index and long-term maintenance treatment. Lancet 1:41, 1977

54. Rybakowski J, Strzyzewski W: Red-blood-cell lithium index and long-term maintenance treatment. Lancet 1:1408−1409, 1976

55. Sacchetti E, Bottinelli S, Bellodi L, et al: Erythrocyte/plasma lithium ratios. Lancet 1:908, 1977

56. von Knorring L, Oreland L, Perris C, et al: Lithium RBC/plasma ratio in subgroups of patients with affective disorders. Neuropsychobiology 2:74−80, 1976

57. Ehrlich BE, Diamond JM: An ultramicro method for analysis of lithium and other biologically important cations. Biochem et Biophys Acta 543:264−268, 1978

58. Spitzer RL, Endicott J, Robins E: Research Diagnostic Criteria (RDC) for a Selected Group of Functional Disorders. NIMH Clinical Research Branch, or contact Drs. Spitzer and Endicott, Biometrics Research, NY State Psychiatric Institute, NY NY

59. Cade JFL: Lithium: past, present and future, in FN Johnson and S Johnson (eds): Lithium in Medical Practice. Baltimore, University Park Press, 1978, p 9

Jeffery N. Wilkins

6
Neuroendocrinology and Clinical Psychiatry

Geoffrey Harris provided the thrust for modern neuroendocrinology by recognizing the vast implications of brain-pituitary connections in hormone regulation.[1] This established the background for investigators to define the hypothalamic-pituitary vocabulary and syntax. The first key substrate to be identified and synthesized was the three amino acid peptide, thyrotropin-releasing-hormone (TRH).[2,3] Pioneer investigators R. Guillemin and A. Schally shared the Nobel prize for this and related work in 1977. It is now known that small peptides frequently serve as primary releasing or inhibiting messengers from the hypothalamus to the pituitary.

Technical advances have accelerated the growth of neuroendocrinology. Perhaps the most significant advance is the radioimmunoassay developed by Yalow and Berson in 1960 which allows accurate measurement of peptide and steroid hormones in body fluids.[4] Two excellent reviews of the evolution of neuroendocrinology and its contributors have been published by Ganong and Martini,[5] and Zimmerman et al.[6]

Neuroendocrine studies are rapidly gaining significance in many areas of medicine. In clinical psychiatry neuroendocrine hormones have been implicated in the physiology of stress, the schizophrenic and depressive disorders, anorexia nervosa, psychosocial dwarfism, some psychosexual disorders, and premenstrual syndromes. Studies of hormonal release patterns in humans suggest altered secretion in psychopathologic states as well as in response to treatment. Comprehensive reviews on neuroendocrines, psychopathology and psychopharmacology are available from Sachar et al[7] and Carroll.[8] This selective review focuses on neuroendocrine studies in schizophrenic and depressive disorders.

SCHIZOPHRENIC DISORDERS

Snyder has proposed that one likely neural substrate for a "locus of schizophrenia" is the mesolimbic dopamine (DA) system.[9] Neuroleptics have been shown to block central nervous system (CNS) DA receptors[10] and can produce side effects of pseudoparkinsonism, akinesia and tardive dyskinesia, all of which may be due to drug-induced dysfunction of DA activity in the nigrostriatum.[11]

In man, mesolimbic DA activity can be studied indirectly through cerebrospinal fluid determinations of total DA metabolism. However, the mesolimbic DA network is one of seven central DA systems and contributes a minor fraction to total CNS DA turnover. By contrast, the nigrostriatum accounts for approximately eighty per cent of the total.[12]

Blood prolactin is an accessible and quantifiable substrate whose release may reflect mesolimbic DA activity. Prolactin is tonically inhibited by DA activity of the tuberoinfundibulum,[13] a network similar in structure and physiology to the mesolimbic DA system.[14] To date, most investigations of prolactin in schizophrenia have focused on three pragmatic questions: (1) Will baseline levels of prolactin differentiate unmedicated schizophrenic patients from control subjects? (2) Do all effective neuroleptics result in blood prolactin elevations? (3) Does the blood prolactin concentration parallel blood neuroleptic levels? Selected studies discussed below address these questions. The first two issues are largely resolved while findings on the third are as yet inconclusive.

Meltzer et al, in a study of 22 newly admitted unmedicated schizophrenic patients, found that normals and schizophrenics had similar patterns of basal and chlorpromazine-stimulated blood prolactin (Fig. 6-1).[15] These investigators concluded that the hypothesized disturbance in brain dopamine in schizophrenia appears not to extend to the tuberoinfundibulum. Yet, though basal prolactin levels are not affected by schizophrenia, extending the above study to include repeated measures of prolactin following neuroleptic challenge would increase the chances for differentiating schizophrenic patients from controls.

Thus far, investigations on all effective antipsychotic drugs have shown that they share the ability to block dopamine receptors[16] and stimulate prolactin release in humans.[17] However, are the prolactin-releasing effects of the neuroleptics separable from clinical responsivity? Investigations of the neuroleptic clozapine have addressed this question. Clozapine is an effective neuroleptic lacking pseudoparkinsonian side effects and is, therefore, believed not to block DA receptors in the nigrostriatum. Sachar initially reported that clozapine resulted only in minor drug-induced prolactin elevations in humans.[7] Following this study, Meltzer demonstrated significant elevations of

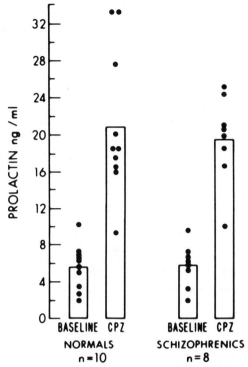

Fig. 6-1. Plasma prolactin concentrations before and 2 hr after i.m. administration of 25 mg chlorpromazine in normal and schizophrenic men. (Reprinted, with permission, from Sachar EJ: Neuroendocrine responses to psychotropic drugs, in Lipton MA, Dimascio A, Killam KF (eds): Psychopharmacology: A Generation of Progress. New York, Raven Press, 1978, p 501.)

prolactin in humans following clozapine administration, though high doses were required.[18] On the basis of these findings it cannot be claimed that the clozapine effect contradicts the neuroleptic-prolacting stimulation paradigm; however, the clozapine studies do indicate physiological separation of neuroleptic blockage of DA activity in the basal ganglia from DA blockage in the tuberoinfundibular tract.

Drug blood levels of tricyclic antidepressants and lithium are routine clinical measures in the psychopharmacologic treatment of depression.[19] The usefulness of neuroleptic drug levels in the treatment of schizophrenia is being tested by numerous investigators. If prolactin responses prove to correlate with drug levels, then prolactin measures may substitute for the more complex and expensive drug analyses.

Dose-response comparisons of neuroleptic-induced prolactin elevations demonstrate a plateau of prolactin within the first few hours, frequently at dosages below the theraeutic range. Therefore, meaningful correlates between drug and prolactin levels would occur prior to this saturation effect. Kaul and Sachar have demonstrated a positive correlation ($r = .81$) of plasma prolactin with chlorpromazine (CPZ) levels following a 25 mg CPZ challenge (Fig. 6-2).[20] They report that about 65 percent of the variance among subjects in prolactin response to the standard dose can be accounted for by differences in blood drug level. Therefore, within a selective range, the degree of prolactin enhancement parallels the relative clinical potencies of neuroleptics.

The parallel between prolactin stimulation and neuroleptic potency

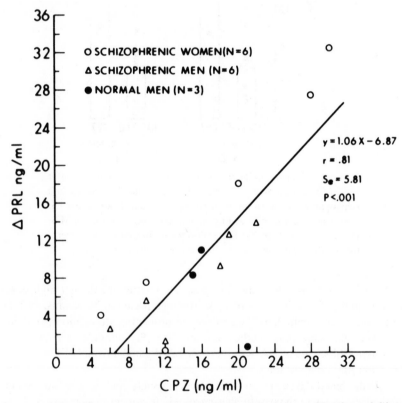

Fig. 6-2. Correlation between plasma prolactin increases at 60 min and blood chlorpromazine concentration at 45 min after i.m. 25 mg chlorpromazine. (Reprinted, with permission, from Sachar EJ: Neuroendocrine responses to psychotropic drugs, in Lipton MA, Dimascio A, Killam KF (eds): Psychopharmacology: A Generation of Progress. New York, Raven Press, 1978, p 503.)

suggests the use of prolactin measures as an index of clinical efficacy of the neuroleptics. Depot neuroleptics, which are used most often in the treatment of schizophrenic disorders, can be monitored for continuing effect by prolactin measures. Drug effect is reflected in prolactin stimulation (Fig. 6-3). In keeping with this, a number of investigations have suggested use of routine prolactin measures to monitor drug compliance in patients treated with these agents.

The neuroleptic-prolactin model is not free of discrepancies; leaders in the field have cited a number of problems. Clozapine has a weak prolactin effect, in contrast to its significant clinical effect. In addition, there are a number of chemical agents which increase blood prolactin but lack neuroleptic activity.[21] Other clinical discrepancies exist as well. The prolactin response to neuroleptics is immediate yet the antipsychotic effects of the neuroleptics may be delayed by days or weeks. Discontinuation of the drug results in the return of prolactin to baseline within 2 to 4 days while the antipsychotic effect remains long beyond this time period.[10]

Despite the discrepancies listed, the evidence is compelling for prolactin to be tried as a potentially valuable marker in the treatment of schizophrenia. The prolactin response to neuroleptic treatment may eventually assist the psychopharmacologist in testing the dopamine theory of schizophrenia and may ultimately prove clinically useful as an index of neuroleptic dosage and drug effect.

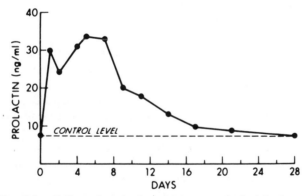

Fig. 6-3.   Prolonged prolactin response to a single injection of depot fluphenazine enanthate 10 mg i.m. in a woman diagnosed as schizoaffective. (Reprinted, with permission, from Sachar EJ, Gruen PH, Altman N. Halpern FS, Frantz AG: The use of neuroendocrine techniques in psychopharmacological research, in Sachar EJ (ed): Hormones, Behavior, and Psychopathology. New York, Raven Press, 1976, p 173.)

CASE EXAMPLES

May and Van Putten have reported on CPZ plasma and saliva "test dose response" in schizophrenic patients.[22] Prolactin measures in these same plasma samples are part of a collaborative effort at the Brentwood Veteran's Administration Medical Center. Four case examples are presented to demonstrate the potential of prolactin measures in differentiating clinical subtypes of schizophrenic patients.

Acute prolactin responses in two subjects to a challenge oral dose of 50 mg CPZ are seen in Figure 6-4. Substantial elevations of prolactin following CPZ administration are seen in both subjects. Differences in the slope (or rate) of prolactin response, and differences in peak response, are evident. Two explanations for the variation in prolactin response are differences in drug availability to the tuberoinfundibulum and individual variation in responsivity of the tuberoinfundibular tract to DA blockage.

Figures 6-5 and 6-6 demonstrate the temporal correlations of plasma prolactin and plasma and saliva CPZ in two subjects. Plasma prolactin, and plasma and saliva CPZ, parallel in subject C over time (hours to weeks). In subject D, prolactin parallels salivary CPZ more closely than plasma CPZ, though not at all points. Although the mechanisms for such individual differences is unclear, the hope is that such variation will correlate with the patient's outcome response to the drug.

DEPRESSIVE DISORDERS

The most extensively studied endocrine axis in endogenous depression is the hypothalamic-pituitary-adrenocortical (HPA) axis. Studies have focused on cortisol metabolism, tissue levels of cortisol, the regulatory mechanisms of cortisol secretion, and the cortisol response to dexamethasone. Two recent reviews on these studies have been published by B. Carroll and J. Mendels.[23,24]

The most consistent and probably most significant disruption of HPA activity in depressed patients is the loss of circadian rhythmicity. Plasma cortisol levels in depressed patients are much higher than control levels, with an attendant loss of normal diurnal variation. Carroll reported that in six depressed patients the mean cortisol production rate was 30.1 mg/day, and fell to a mean of 19.7 mg/day on recovery. The mean production rate for eight control subjects was 17.2 mg/day.[23]

In similar studies, Sachar has found nocturnal hypersecretion of cortisol[25] while Carroll and Mendels demonstrated a loss or early release from dexamethasone suppression in approximately half of the subjects tested (Fig. 6-7).

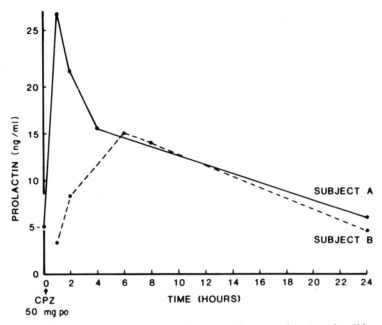

Fig. 6-4. Plasma prolactin response to 50 mg po chlorpromazine "test dose" in two schizophrenic men. (From unpublished data of Wilkins JN, Carlson HJ, VanPutten T, May PRA: Plasma prolactin relationships to plasma and saliva chlorpromazine levels in schizophrenic patients.)

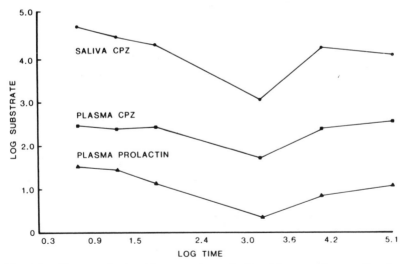

Fig. 6-5. Plasma prolactin, chlorpromazine and saliva chlorpromazine over time in a schizophrenic subject. (From unpublished data of Wilkins JN, Carlson HJ, VanPutten T, May PRA: Plasma prolactin relationships to plasma and saliva chlorpromazine levels in schizophrenic patients.)

107

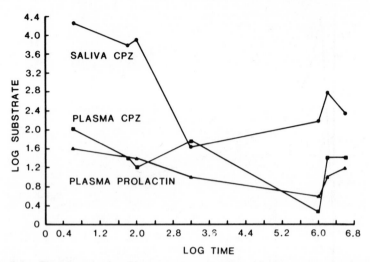

Fig. 6-6.   Plasma prolactin, chlorpromazine and saliva chlorpromazine over time in a schizophrenic subject. (From unpublished data of Wilkins JN, Carlson HJ, VanPutten T, May PRA: Plasma prolactin relationships to plasma and saliva chlorpromazine levels in schizophrenic patients.)

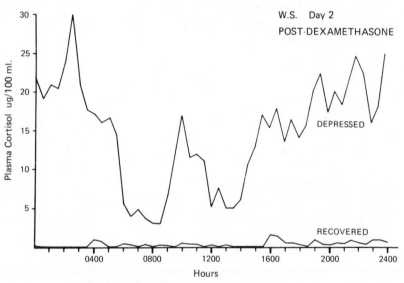

Fig. 6–7.   Plasma cortisol concentrations following dexamethasone 2 mg po in a depressed patient studied before and after treatment. Blood samples were obtained every 30 min through a venous catheter. Dexamethasone was given at midnight on each occasion. (Reprinted, with permission, from Carroll BJ, Mendels J: Neuroendocrine regulation in affective disorders, in Sachar EG (ed): Hormones, Behavior, and Psychopathology. New York, Raven Press, p 208.)

Other hormones under study in depression are thyrotropin releasing hormone[24] and growth hormone. Langer et al recently reported on human growth hormone (HGH) response to a single intravenous administration of amphetamine sulfate (0.1 mg/kg) in control subjects and in patients diagnosed as having reactive depression, endogenous depression, schizophrenia, or chronic alcoholism. All patients were tested during overt manifestations of their disease. Peak levels of HGH were obtained between 30 and 60 minutes following the intravenous amphetamine injection. Compared with the control subjects, endogenously depressed patients released significantly less HGH ($p < .01$) and patients with reactive depression significantly more HGH ($p < 0.5$). Human growth hormone response to intravenous amphetamine in the patients with schizophrenia and chronic alcoholism did not significantly differ from that of the control subjects.[27]

In summary, neuroendocrine hormone measures are useful tools in the diagnosis and ongoing evaluation of patients with depression. Basal cortisol levels and cortisol responses to dexamethasone suppression have proven themselves as valuable adjuncts in the diagnosis of severe depression and as markers of clinical recovery. The less studied growth hormone response to amphetamine challenge may serve to distinguish endogenous depression from reactive depression.

CONCLUSION

Both psychiatric clinicians and investigators will have interest in studies implicating neuroendocrine hormones as markers for major psychiatric syndromes. Dysfunctional neural substrates for psychiatric disease states may alter brain-hormone control mechanisms. The clinician might use neuroendocrine markers for assistance in diagnosis, selection of treatment, and evaluation of treatment outcome. The investigator may wish to unravel complex neurotransmitter-hormone interplay in the hopes of establishing etiologies for mental illness.

Basal plasma cortisol levels and plasma cortisol response to dexamethasone suppression are increasing in use as adjuncts in the diagnosis and treatment of severe depression; the use of stimulated growth hormone response demands further investigation.

Neuroleptic-stimulated prolactin levels in schizophrenic patients are under study in a number of centers. An important task is to identify whether variation between patients in prolactin response to controlled neuroleptic challenge defines subsets of patients who in turn have varying responses to the drug. The same measures might identify which antipsychotic is ideal for a given patient based upon a prolactin response profile.

REFERENCES

1. Harris G: Neural Control of the Pituitary Gland. Baltimore, Williams & Wilkins, 1955
2. Burgus R, Dunn TF, Desiderio D, Guillemin R: Molecular structure of the hypothalamic thyrotropin-releasing factor (TRF) of ovin origin; demonstration of the pyroglutamylhistidylprolinamide sequency by mass spectrometry. Paris, C.R. Acad Sci, (Ser D), 269:1870−1873, 1969
3. Bowers CY, Schally AV, Enzmann F, Boler J, Folkers K: Porcine thyrotropin releasing hormone is (pyro) glu-his-pro (NH2). Endocrinology 86:1143−1153, 1970
4. Yalow RS, Berson SA: Immunoassay of endogenous plasma insulin in man. J Clin Invest 39:1157−1175, 1960
5. Ganong WF, Martini L: Frontiers in Neuroendocrinology. New York, Oxford University Press, 1973
6. Zimmerman E, Gispen WH, Marks BH, DeWied D: Drug Effects on Neuroendocrine Regulation Progress in Brain Research (vol. 39). Amsterdam, Elsevier, 1973
7. Sachar EJ, Gruen PH, Altman N, Halpern FS, Frantz AG: The use of neuroendocrine techniques in psychopharmacological research, in E J Sachar (ed): Hormones, Behavior, and Psychopathology. New York, Raven Press, 1976, pp 161−176
8. Carroll BJ: Neuroendocrine function in psychiatric disorders in Psychopharmacology, Lipton M A, Dimascio A, Killam K F (eds): A Generation of Progress. New York, Raven Press, 1978, pp 487−498
9. Snyder SH, Banerjee SP, Yamamura HI, Greenberg D: Drugs, neurotransmitters and schizophrenia. Science 184:1243−1253, 1974
10. Gruen PH, Sachar EJ, Langer G, Altman N, Liefer M, Frantz A, Halpern FS: Prolactin responses to neuroleptics in normal and schizophrenic subjects. Arch Gen Psychiat 35(1):108−116, 1978
11. Sachar EJ, Gruen PH, Altman N, Liefer M, Halpern FS: Prolactin response to neuroleptic drugs: An approach to the study of brain dopamine blockade, In Usdin E, Hamburg DA, Barchas JS (eds): Neuroregulators and Psychiatric Disorders. New York, Oxford University Press, 1977, pp 242−249
12. Anden NE, Dahlstrom A, Fuxe K, Lavsson K, Olson L, Ungertedt U: Ascending monamine neurons to the telecephalon and diencephalon. Acta Physiol Scand 67:313−326, 1966
13. Meites J: Evaluation of research on control of prolactin secretion. Adv Exp Med Biol 80:135−152, 1977
14. MacLeod R, Lehmeyer JE: Studies on the mechanism of the dopamine-mediated inhibition of prolactin secretion. Endocrinology 94:1077−1085, 1974
15. Meltzer HY, Sachar EJ, Frantz AG: Serum prolactin levels in unmedicated schizophrenic patients. Arch Gen Psychiat 31:564−569, 1974
16. Matthysse S: Antipsychotic drug actions: A clue to the neuropathology of schizophrenia. Fed Proc 32:2, 200−205, 1973
17. Langer G, Sachar EJ, Halpern FS, Gruen PH, Solomon M: The prolactin

response to neuroleptic drugs. A test of dopaminergic blockade: Neuroendocrine studies in normal men. J Clin Endocr Metab 45(5):996–1002, 1977

18. Meltzer HY, Daniels S, Fang VS: Clozapine increases rat serum prolactin levels. Life Sci 17:339–342, 1975

19. Davis JM: Overview: Maintenance therapy in psychiatry: II. Affective disorders. Am J Psychiat 133(1):1–13, 1976

20. Sachar EJ: Neuroendocrine responses to psychotropic drugs, in Lipton MA, Dimascio A, Killam KF (eds): Psychopharmacology: A Generation of Progress. New York, Raven Press, 1978, pp 499–508

21. Turkington RW: Prolactin secretion in patients treated with various drugs. Arch Intern Med 130:349–354, 1972

22. May PRA, Van Putten T, Jenden DJ, Cho AK: Test dose response in schizophrenia. Arch Gen Psychiat 35:1091–1097, 1978

23. Carroll BJ, Curtis GC, Mendels J: Neuroendocrinology regulation in depression. Arch Gen Psychiat 33:1051–1057, 1976

24. Carroll BJ, Mendels J: Neuroendocrine regulation in affective disorders, In Sachar EG (ed): Hormones, Behavior, and Psychopathology. New York, Raven Press, 1976, pp 193–224

25. Sachar EJ, Hellman L, Roffwarg HP, et al: Disrupted 24-hour patterns of cortisol secretion in psychotic depression. Arch Gen Psychiat 28:19–24, 1973

26. Langer G, Heinze G, Reim R, Matussek N: Reduced growth hormone responses to amphetamine in "endogenous" depressive patients. Arch Gen Psychiat 33:1471–1475, 1976

PART III

Interactional Themes

Milton Greenblatt

Introduction

How does psychiatric research enlighten psychiatric practice? Every practitioner is anxious to be as fully up-to-date as possible, to take advantage of every bit of new knowledge that could have practical therapeutic value. And what is most useful? For some practitioners, new concepts that help to explain behavioral phenomena are very important. Witness how much the understanding of human emotions has been enlightened by Freudian psychodynamics. For other practitioners, any new light shed upon specific mechanisms of disease is highly appreciated. But for all practitioners, any new treatment approach, and practical avenue of help for the troubled patients, is eagerly sought.

Throughout this book and particularly in the chapters of this section, which Dr. Serafetinides has aptly labeled "Interactional Themes," we find insights, concepts and investigative results that will be of help to many practitioners. Interactional themes are found in the subtle interplay of biological, psychological and social factors, both in etiology and in treatment approaches. Each author is fully aware that no individual, and certainly no sick individual, is less than the sum of these considerations. Despite the complexity, progress is being made.

In Pasnau's chapter on Psychosomatic Medicine, two highly useful therapeutic modes are presented. One has to do with an holistic approach to the treatment of breast cancer, in which the victim and her family are sensitively conducted through a deep educational and therapeutic experience that starts at the moment when the dread diagnosis is made, and is carried through the period of surgery as well as postoperative rehabilitation. Breast cancer is not merely a tragedy limited to the female affected; it involves all the family and significant others. Only the broadest view of management will in the future be accepted as adequate medical care.

Pasnau then reviews the comforting work of Rahe, which proposes that group therapy with post myocardial infarction patients probably prevents recurrences and increases survival time. How revealing of the broad psychosocial significance of the coronary event. Surely, this new discovery deserves trial everywhere, with the hope that the apparent good results may be improved further.

Yager, Rudnick, and Metzner's review of Anorexia Nervosa is not only authorative and comprehensive, but their explanation of the meaning of body image to patients, as revealed by direct confrontation through television and via specific questioning regarding satisfaction with their general morphology (as well as specific parts), is a new and promosing approach to the understanding of the socio-psychopathology of anorectic disease. The general management of anorexia, as described in their experience, again requires a complex socio-psychological reward-type step system that ought to receive further trial and confirmation in other settings.

Hiroto and Peters' vivid analysis of learned helplessness, and its analogy to classical depression, opens up a new way of thinking about this disorder. Hiroto's personal investigative contributions to this problem are impressive. Seeing depression as a series of losses due to uncontrollable forces, and interpreted by the patient as due to his or her inadequacy, with consequent negative effect on self-esteem, is certainly an interesting way to think about this ancient illness. The studies quoted help to identify the specific sensitive points in the mechanisms of this complicated illness and also to rationalize some of the cognitive therapeutic approaches that have become popular lately.

Finally, Pope's highly original analysis of how and why research has tended to shy away from some of the most important issues in psychotherapy, sets up thinking on a new set of problems. Concerning the desirability of charging healthy fees in order to keep patients working seriously on their problems, Pope gives us evidence that the way Freud and some of the pioneering psychoanalysts have viewed this problem is not necessarily convincing today. These and other clinical issues he treats with amusing penetration.

Robert O. Pasnau

7
Psychosomatic Medicine

THE PSYCHOSOMATIC APPROACH

In his brilliantly conceived and written book Psychobiology and Human Disease (1977) Weiner has described the comprehensive view of disease known as the "psychosomatic approach." It is based on the fundamental observation that persons are more than the sum of the cells and organ systems of which they are constituted, and that it is persons who have diseases. It follows that the psychosomatic approach involves appreciation of genetic contributions, immune mechanisms, social environments, cultural settings, educational and nutritional experiences, exposure to toxic and infectious agents, and physiological and psychological development. How these various factors interact and result in the failure to adapt, which is known as disease, is the subject of psychosomatic research. In most cases, the mechanisms are unknown.[1]

Because of the mystery surrounding the field, as well as the lack of agreement of medical scientists as to the validity of the psychosomatic approach (as Weiner observes, most physicians do not accept the fundamental assumption upon which it is based), the clinical practice of psychosomatic medicine is fraught with many difficulties. Added to the inherent difficulty was the promise of the psychosomatic movement of the 1940s and 1950s which led to expectations of psychiatry and psychoanalysis which could not be fulfilled. Once disillusioned, many young physicians (now senior and often with authority roles in their fields) harbor antagonism towards the latter-day practitioners of the psychosomatic approach (known as consultation liaison psychiatrists), and influence their students in a likewise negative fashion. As a result, much of the current preoccupation of clinical psychosomaticists has been with the systems problem, i.e. how to overcome the many resistances which prevent the application of a psychosomatic approach to patients.[2]

A subject as large and engrossing as this one cannot be captured in a short chapter. The complexity of the research problems is enormous. We are not even at the level of certainty of diagnosis which permits differentiation of types of illness into subclassifications, nor can we specify personality variables except in the most inexact terms. The role of the brain in the mediation and control of each bodily organ is poorly understood, even though each organ system is controlled and regulated by hormones, neural input, immune mechanisms, nutrients, and even volitional and experiential adaptations. Therefore this chapter can serve only as a kind of introduction to the subject and an outline of the clinical areas which seem to be the most promising in terms of impact on patient care. It will touch on the history of psychosomatic concepts, the personality and illness, the precipitation of illness, problems of transduction of stress, consulting with physically ill patients, and clinical research in the area of recuperation and rehabilitation.

THE PERSISTANCE OF HISTORICAL PSYCHOSOMATIC THEORIES

In order to appreciate the modern clinical practice of psychosomatic medicine, the contributions from the past must be understood. In the psychosomatic theories of the past are to be found the roots of most current research and theory.

Throughout recorded history, the basic approach to medicine has been psychosomatic. Practicing physicians have held the belief that the influence of the body and the influence of the mind were inseparable and that one must treat the patient rather than the illness. It is also believed that primitive man held a psychosomatic orientation to illness, i.e. that disease was caused by spiritual powers and must be fought by spiritual means. The evil spirit which enters and affects the total being must be liberated through exorcism or trepanation.[3]

Many patients still hold very primitive beliefs about the causation of illness even in this day of modern medicine. It is not uncommon to find some patients who hold these beliefs consciously; in many other patients these beliefs are lurking closely beneath the surface. Modern physicians often attempt to reassure their patients through methods not unlike the physician priests 10,000 years earler, employing magical treatments to bring about relief of suffering.

During the period between 2500 and 500 B.C., medicine was dominated by religion, but was psychosomatic in all its aspects; suggestion was the main tool of treatment. Similarly, today, many people believe that sin leads to illness and death and that cleansing one's soul is the required catharsis for expiating the sin. Faith healers, using suggestion and belief in divine intervention, attract thousands of followers at each meeting. Even Freud noted that psychoanalysts could hardly compare the letters from a few grateful patients to the millions of cures at Lourdes.[4]

Greek medicine was largely holistic. Hippocrates is credited with the statement, "in order to cure the human body, it is necessary to have a knowledge of the whole." Plato wrote that Socrates said "As it is not proper to cure the eyes without the head nor the head without the body, so neither is it proper to cure the body without the soul." These concepts play a very important role in the practice of psychosomatic medicine today, even though the term "holistic" has become a motto for the avant garde (often antimedical groups) who look to health enhancement, sound living, good diet, exercise, and stress reduction as an answer to the prevention of most illness, including cancer.[5]

In the late Roman civilization, there emerged an individual whose influence on medicine was to extend for a thousand years. He was the Greek slave-physician Galen, whose holistic approach to medicine was combined with an understanding of the natural course of illness. His description of circular insanity is one of the earliest recorded descriptions of bi-polar affective disorder. Galen's humoral theory postulated that disease is caused by disturbance in the fluids of the body. He taught that the major contribution the doctor could make to understanding disease was to observe his patients over a period of time, basing observations on the emotional as well as the physical state of the patient. He described the case of a young woman who came into his consulting room with a rather severe anxiety attack. As he talked with her, she calmed down. It was his habit to continue to monitor the patient's pulse while conducting his interview. As he began to discuss the current events of the day, including the appearance at a local theater of one of the leading male actors of the time, the patient's pulse markedly accellerated. He repeated this procedure during several subsequent appointments, each time talking about a different actor, without the same results. At the end of the week, he proclaimed her a victim of love-sickness and prescribed the appropriate remedy.

The role of psychophysiological assessment of patients is quite important today, as is the role of stress in the precipitation of illness. Much of the research in the past decade has involved the relationship between life events and illness and the reactions of individuals to stress.[6] Also important have been the role of biofeedback in the treatment of psychosomatic disorders and the role of behavior modification in treating patients with psychophysiological disorders.[7,8]

Between 500 A.D. and 1600 A.D. there was a reemergence of the mystical with the religious domination of medicine. The belief was that sinning was the cause of all degenerative illnesses, and of mental illnesses in particular. This was also the time of the religious cures, with burning being the primary method for curing people with mental illness. Torture and various forms of deprivation were also employed. The persistence of this belief is impressive. The belief that masturbation leads to mental illness was widespread in the 19th century. Hundreds of women were castrated in the late 19th century for "incurable masturbation."[9] In this century Baden Powell's Handbook for Boys included a warning against "self-abuse"[10] Lipowski writes that the religious belief of illness as punishment is a significant implication of illness to many patients.[11]

Between 1500 and 1800, there was a renewed interest in the natural sciences and their applications to medicine. As an example are the works of the Vesalius in anatomy, and van Leeuwenhoek, whose first exploration using the microscope was to examine his own seminal fluid. Interestingly enough, the psychic influences on the soma were rejected as unscientific, and the study of the mind was taken out of the medical and put into the philosophical arena. A major exception was one of the great physicians of the time, Sydenham, who believed that the disorders known as hysteria and hypochondrias belonged in the medical field.[12] Hysteria was thought to be a disease of women and hypochondriasis a disease of men. This idea has persisted to the present time. It is very unusual to find a male suffering from hysteria even in a V.A. hospital. What is important, however, is that research into hypochondriasis and hysteria have provided some of the most important biobehavioral contributions to the field of psychosomatic medicine, particularly through the observations of Janet, Freud, and later psychoanalytic investigators.

The 19th century marked the end of the psychosomatic approach in medicine. Modern science and modern laboratory medicine progressed, as exemplified by the work of Virchow in Germany. His dictum, that in order to understand pathology one must understand what's happening at the cellular level, marked the beginning of specialization of medicine. By about 1850, the time of the second Viennese medical revolution, medicine began to focus on the individual organ systems and illnesses rather than on the patients. This was the beginning of the great advances in medicine, a time when professors stopped lecturing in Latin and began to lecture in national languages so that medical students easily could understand what they were saying. They also began to make rounds, examining patients personally rather than diagnosing from afar. Before this time most professors of medicine taught from their offices and made their diagnoses without ever seeing the patients, because it was thought to be too dangerous to expose them to whatever contagion was to be found in the hospital.* After 1850, professors became a little bit braver. No doubt as a result of this first-hand contact, all kinds of gadgets were developed, leading to technical advances in physical diagnosis. This was a great revolution in medicine, and medical practice underwent a dramatic change away from the individual patient and toward the illness.

For the first time in the history of medicine, something called ''psychosomatic medicine'' emerged. Prior to this time it was unnecessary to have a psychosomatic medicne; medicine was pcychosomatic. Although Heinroth had used the term psychosomatic in the early 19th century, it was through the writings of Von Feuchtersleben that the first comprehensive psychosomatic approach to medicine was presented.[13] His chairmanship of the Department of Psychiatry at Vienna set an important precedent for those who followed. Psychosomatic medicine was nourished in Vienna even as it was abandoned throughout the rest of the medical world.

Modern psychosomatic medicine is biopsychosocial medicine. It represents an attempt to recapture focus on the patient and to put together all of the factors that influence the individual patient as a person; the social system, the family, the relationships with others as well as the patient's psychological state.[14]

PERSONALITY AND ILLNESS

It is well known in medical practice that about 25 percent of the population experience 75 percent of the illness. This has led to the observations by physicians of individuals who appear to be illness-prone or pain-prone. Osler, in his address to a graduating class in 1910, observed that special personality characteristics were to be found in his patients suffering from coronary heart disease.[15] Dunbar, who was one of the very first to identify herself as a consultation-liaison psychiatrist, was equally impressed by the apparent association of personality and illness. She hypothesized that there were specific personality profiles of individuals prone to develop certain organic diseases. She was one of the first to use the term ''coronary-prone personality''. She believed that various psychosomatic illnesses occurred in specific personality types.[16]

Alexander also emphasized the characterologic features of patients suffering from specific psychosomatic disorders, even though he differed

---

*An interesting observation is that much psychiatric training takes place in the fashion of pre-1850; that is, the supervisor rarely sees the patient that the resident is treating, and makes all of his diagnoses from afar.

somewhat from Dunbar. He found that individuals who were basically passive and dependent but had been thrust into unwanted positions of responsibility and leadership often developed symptoms of peptic ulcers. He believed that chronic hypersecretion of gastric juices was an expression of ongoing unfulfilled infantile longings. To him the asthmatic attack represented a cry for help from a child to a basically unloving mother and was a somatic expression of an underlying depression. He also believed that poorly controlled conflicts over the recognition and expression of aggression in circumstances which would, under normal circumstances, provoke rage or hostility, led to the development of arterial hypertension. Similar speculations about dermatological disorders and ulcerative colitis were offered, and attempts were made to validate these speculations and observations through the use of psychoanalytic techniques and projective psychological testing.[17]

Alexander differed from Freud in stressing that psychosomatic symptoms were not symbolic of unconscious psychic elaborations which were found in neurotic patients, but that they appeared to be the result of chronic autonomic activity associated with repressed affects that could not be discharged to the normal overt expression of the emotion. He differentiated between hysterical conversion, and psychosomatic conditions, which he called vegetative neuroses. He described vegetative neurosis as a psychogenic dysfunction of a vegetative organ which was not under control of voluntary neuromuscular system. Although at the present time the distinction between conversion and psychosomatic symptoms no longer is as clearcut, Alexander's observations and experimentations were extremely influential in shaping the course of psychosomatic research.

Linn points out that Alexander's contributions to clinical psychosomatic practice emphasized the importance of an individual approach to each patient, underscoring the need to assess individual intrapsychic conflicts in order to understand the precipitation of the illness, the form of the illness, the eventual recovery, and therapeutic strategies for the patient. However, the initial hope for the discovery of specific personality factors in illness was frustrated by the failure to accurately differentiate forms of illness, and the unfortunate tendency to lump such entities as peptic ulcer or bronchial asthma or hypertension into single categories despite the fact that these categories represent a wide spectrum of etiological and pathophysiological disorders.[18]

Perhaps the most important current contribution to the research in personality factors in illness has been the work of Friedman and Rosenman with the "Type A personality". Following the work of Osler and Dunbar, they described the individual who was most likely to develop coronary illness as over-controlled, over-conscientious, working against the clock, either as a workaholic or a sisyphus, i.e. an individual who is continually unsatisfied with his or her performance. These people are less likely to be flexible at times of stress. In those who are also predisposed genetically or by environment to develop coronary disease, they are 8 times more likely to develop coronary illness in the fifth decade than their non-Type A peer control group, and about 2½ times more likely to develop coronary illness in their sixth decade.[19] It should be stressed, however, that while this enhancement is statistically significant, nonetheless most Type A personalities do not develop coronary illness.

At the present time, the clinical practitioner of the psychosomatic approach is impressed by the importance of personality factors in illness. It is clear that personality is deeply rooted in the life experiences of the individual, and may have a contribution from genetic factors such as mood or disposition. At the same time, it is clear that there is an interaction between personality factors and the environmental factors. Certain behaviors may be rewarded or punished by important persons in the environment. At the same time, the life pattern which we call personality, is only one part of the psychosomatic process. The factors of daily living with its stresses and life change and the biological predisposition to illness are equally important parts of the equation that may result in one patient developing an illness and in the other, successful coping and health.

THE PRECIPITATION OF ILLNESS

Engel and his coworkers have shown that a generalized sense of loss (either actual, potential, or imaginary) and bereavement are significant factors in the onset of most diseases. They have found that feelings of loss lead to a complex emotional response of hopelessness and helplessness. This in turn results in an adaptive psychological failure during which the individual can no longer cope with environmental tasks.[20]

It is generally accepted today that the decision to visit a doctor is the result not only of the abnormality within the patient but also of life changes to which the patient can not adapt. This finding is the major contribution of Holmes and Rahe, who have listed the commonly encountered life changes and have attempted to quantitate the traumatic impact of each event as measured in what they call "life change units". For example, according to their scale, the death of a spouse has an impact value of 100, and going on vacation a value of 13. According to their findings, the accumulation of over 200 life change units in a year is associated with a high incident of illness.[21] Unconscious factors may be as important as are conscious factors. For example, during a period of stress an individual is considered to be more accident prone or illness prone. Long ignored symptoms of illness may receive new attention and the decision to seek medical help for ignored symptoms may signal the failure of the adaptation process to life stress. It has been consistently observed that individuals who are undergoing significant life changes are more vulnerable to injuries, accidents and illnesses of all kinds. It is not surprising that children's visits to the pediatrician correspond to parental periods of stress. Not only are childhood symptoms accentuated during periods of parental stress, but it is also observed that parents who find it difficult to control their own disruptive impulses use emergency rooms as ways of dealing with unacceptable destructive impulses toward their children. Traumatic life changes may precipitate disease involving any organ system of the body with any degree of severity. In addition, it may lead to symptoms without organic disease, or renewed concerns about old or ignored illness, or any combination of the above.

The renewed focus on family practice has also served to emphasize the observation that illness which appears to be an individual one can really be the expression of the family disturbance. One of the major contributions of Masters and Johnson has been their insistence that the treatment of the sexual dysfunction in one marital partner involves the couple and not the individual alone.[22] Not only may one marital partner become ill when illness occurs in the house, but it has been repeatedly demonstrated that widows and widowers are more likely to deteriorate physically and die during the bereavement periods than nonwidowed peer controls.[23]

Thus, research has shown that the understanding of the psychosocial milieu in which the illness develops, as well as an understanding of the current life situation and dramatic life changes which have occurred in the preceding period, are crucial to understanding why illness develops in a particular patient at a particular time.

THE TRANSDUCTION OF STRESS

Even though clinicians have known for centuries that stressful situations precede the development of illness, most researchers have not studied the mechanisms through which the stressful experience is translated or transduced into somatic responses. Alexander's observation that the patients suffering from psychosomatic disorders appear to handle the psychological experiences in a different manner from normal neurotics, began an interesting and useful area of research into the intrapsychic differences that some of these individuals demonstrate.

In 1960 Marty and de M'Uzan, two French psychoanalysts, described what they called "pensee operatoire" in patients suffering from psychosomatic disorders. They defined this as thought content characterized by a preoccupation with the minutia of their daily lives.[24] Shortly thereafter, Sifneos coined the term "alexithymia," observing that psychosomatic patients are often unable to describe their feelings in words (no words for feelings).[25] This term and the observation struck a responsive note with clinicians working in clinical psychosomatic medicine, and much attention has been paid to this phenomenon. (It should be noted that it occurs in some, but not all, patients with psychosomatic disorders.) The difficulty in verbalization does not appear to be related to educational level or intelligence. Nemiah has described the case of the individual who recognizes that "I can not put my feelings into words". In addition to the verbal deficit, they are often unable to localize common somatic reactions that usually accompany the experience of a variety of emotions. Many appear to be unable to distinguish between anger, anxiety, grief, and happiness. All affects appear to be experienced equally in an undifferentiated fashion. Another striking observation is that they are unable to recount fantasies about their affectual life, and they are unable to recall dreams. Their speech lacks emotional coloring. Alexithymia in addition to pensee operatoire results in a rather boring interview. Many physicians find these patients intolerable, difficult and frustrating. Nemiah differentiates these individuals from obsessional patients. In the former, both affect and fantasy are affected. In the latter there is an extensive and often incredible repertoire of conscious fantasies which are readily available for the therapy or analysis.[26]

Hoppe has described a group of individuals with alexithymia who have survived Nazi concentration camp experiences. Some 30 to 50 percent subsequently developed psychosomatic illnesses. He believes that the psychosomatic reactions in these patients represent a regression from a more mature affective level to a more primitive one. He postulates a return to developmentally earlier channels of expression in which feelings are diffusely discharged into the body without symbolization. This has been termed the resomatization theory of psychosomatic medicine.[27]

This model of symptom production is used by most psychosomatic clinicians and researchers at the present time. Despite differences in the conceptualization of transduction, most believe that environmental stress sets in motion an aroused internal state in an individual subjected to the stress, and that the arousal, instead of finding an outlet via the channels, which in normals or neurotics lead to affective fantasy, is discharged directly into channels affecting bodily functioning.

It is clear that the etiology of psychosomatic disorders is a complicated matter. No single theoretical model suffices to explain all of the clinical observations. Furthermore, not all patients with psychosomatic disorders suffer from or are observed to have the condition known as alexithymia.

Nonetheless, research has shown that there are differences in the coping mechanisms and psychodynamics of patients with primary psychosomatic disorders.

CONSULTING WITH PHYSICALLY ILL PATIENTS AND THEIR PHYSICIANS

Lipowski, who is the contemporary spokesman for liaison psychiatry, has described the three primary functions of consultation-liaison psychiatry. These are: clinical service, which includes diagnostic as well as therapeutic intervention; teaching; and research. The major tactics of the current model emphasize the role of prevention, and the need for a close relationship between the treating physician and the consulting psychiatrist.[28] Over the years in many hospitals, psychiatric units have developed with their affiliated consultation-liaison programs. Close collaboration with the nurses and other members of the health care team leads to psychosocial conferences in which patients are discussed with other members of the treatment team. Consultation to patients then flows from the observed needs of the patients and their families. Many patients and families who are seen for preventive work are brought very early into the treatment planning process.

Usually underemphasized in the current liaison model is the opportunity for psychotherapeutic interventions with patients. Wahl has pointed out the unique opportunity afforded to the psychiatrist in doing intensive short-term psychotherapy with patients. He has found that the situation of treating patients confined in a hospital affords one the opportunity to do the work that is not paralleled in many hours of outpatient therapy.[29] Schwab and Kuhn have likewise demonstrated the importance of psychotherapy and the resolution of rather significant conflicts in such setting.[30]

The principles of the liaison psychiatry emphasize prevention and close collaboration between physicians. It is psychosomatic in all aspects. The liaison psychiatrist stresses the coexistance of the psychosocial and biological phenomena of health and disease. This orientation is difficult for physicians who have based their view of illness on the long-standing disease oriented approach. It becomes very difficult for these physicians to substitute the patient-oriented or biopsychosocial approach. Nonetheless, without it, the patient is often abandoned to a frighteningly alien technological and de-humanized medical environment.

A major problem for contemporary consultation-liaison psychiatry is the scope of modern medicine. Not only does the consultation-liaison psychiatrist need to feel comfortable in a variety of medical environments, but the demands upon his or her ability to know the current pharmacological agents employed in the variety of medical specialties and their interactions with psychotropic medications often leads to frustration. One of the obvious resolutions of this dilemma is to specialize. The past decade has seen the emergence of liaison psychiatric research in a variety of special medical environments and specialities of medicine.[31]

SOMATOPSYCHIC MEDICINE

Psychological reaction to physical illness and the emotional aspects of recovery from illness and rehabilitation are areas in which much contemporary psychiatric research is being undertaken. There is no illness in which psychosocial factors do not account for a large part of the final outcome for the patient and the family. It is not possible to describe in detail the large number of clinical studies which are being conducted in this fascinating area. This section will focus on two studies which can serve as examples of the kind of work which is being done, and highlight the importance of this research to the clinical practice of psychiatry.

The first of these studies was conducted by Pfefferbaum and her associates at UCLA on patients who recently underwent mastectomy. Based upon the findings of their study which looked at the emotional reactions to mastectomy in 41 women patients and their spouses, she devised a program of comprehensive psychosocial care for mastectomy patients which began at the time of the patient's entry into the medical care system and provided follow-up for the difficult rehabilitation and recovery period. Noting that many spouses reported great difficulty in dealing with the physical aspects of mastectomy, including the problems of decreased sexual frequency and unwillingness or inability to view the partner unclothed, support for the spouse was initiated prior to mastectomy and continued throughout the recovery period. Great attention was paid to that particularly stressful period between the diagnosis of cancer and the actual time of mastectomy. Efforts were made to work closely with nursing personnel and helping them deal with their own observed difficulties in treating mastectomy patients. Attention was paid to the teenage children, particularly the teenage daughters of these patients. Noting that over 100,000 American women underwent mastectomy in the past year, and that 33,000 deaths from breast cancer would be expected annually, she pointed to the challenge that breast cancer poses for physicians and for the families of the mastectomy patients. In addition to these problems, patients and family decide whether or not to have breast reconstruction and face the possibility of the spread of the cancer, of recurrence and another mastectomy. This program, which developed out of the findings of a research project, points the way to the use of research in development of programs for psychosocial rehabilitation following traumatic surgery, particularly in cancer patients.[32]

Another example of this kind of research is found in a study of group therapy for myocardial infarction patients. In this study, Rahe and his associates studied a group of myocardial infarction patients for a full year follow-up, using a controlled trial period. Forty-four patients surviving their first MI were randomly allocated to either group therapy, or control group status, and were followed up over a four-year period. An additional 17 patients were referred for group therapy sessions following the termination of the controlled experiment. These patients were also followed for a three-year period. They discovered that patients who received group therapy had significantly less follow-up coronary mortality and morbidity, returned to work at a significantly higher percentage than control patients, and reported a greater quality of their postillness life. Although neither group therapy nor control group patients meaningly altered conventional coronary risk factors (weight, serum colesterol, cigarette smoking), the group therapy patients were able to overcome certain coronary-prone behaviors including overwork and time urgency. It was concluded that the group therapy experience played an important role in determining the rehabilitation advantage that the treated patients had over their nontreated peers. The study also revealed that the treatment of post MI patients is one of great opportunity for the research psychiatrist. The morbidity and mortality data provide hard measurements of therapeutic success, and the return-to-work statistics are more convincing measures of treatment outcome than a patient's report that he is functioning better.[33]

Both of these studies, concerning as they do the number one cancer in women and the number one killer in men, point to the necessity of performing clinical research in the psychosocial aspects of physical illness (somato-psychic medicine). There is a need for a multidisciplinary approach to optimally reduce the toll of death and disability from these major public health problems.

REFERENCES

1. Weiner H: Psychobiology and Human Disease. New York, Elsevier, 1977
2. Krakowski AJ: The process of consultation, in Wittkower ED, Warnes H (eds): Psychosomatic Medicine Its Clinical Applications. Hagerstown, Harper & Row, 1977
3. Kaplan HI: Current psychodynamic concepts in psychosomatic medicine, in Pasnau RO (ed): Consultation-Liaison Psychiatry. New York, Grune & Stratton, 1975

4. Freud S: New introductory lectures in psychoanalysis (1932), in Strachey J (ed & transl): Complete Psychological Works (vol 22). London, Hogarth Press, 1964

5. Simonton CO, Simonton SS: Belief systems and management of the emotional aspects of malignancy. J Transpersonal Psychology 7:29−47, 1975

6. Rahe RH, Arthur RJ: Life changes and illness studies: Past history and future directions. J Human Stress 4:3−15, 1978

7. Shapiro D: Biofeedback, in Pasnau RO (ed): Consultation-Liaison Psychia;ry. New York, Grune & Stratton, 1975

8. Wolpe J: Psychotherapy by Reciprocal Inhibition. Stanford, Stanford University Press, 1958

9. Battey R: Oophorectomy-Battey's operation-spaying-castration of women. Trans Int Med Congr 4:279−288, 1881

10. Baden-Powell R: Handbook for Boys. New York, Boy Scouts of America, 1911

11. Lipowski ZJ: Physical illness, the individual and the coping processes. Psychiatry Med 1:91−102, 1970

12. Veith I: Hysteria: The History of a Disease. Chicago, University of Chicago Press, 1965

13. Von Feuchtersleben E: The principles of medical psychology, in Lloyd HE and Babington BG (eds & transl) London, Sydenham Society, 1847

14. Engel G: The need for a new medical model: A challenge for biomedicine. Science 196:129−135, 1977

15. Osler W: The Lumleian lectures. Lancet 1:839−844, 1910

16. Dunbar HF: Psychosomatic Diagnosis. New York, Hoeber, 1943

17. Alexander F: Psychosomatic Medicine. New York, W.W. Norton, 1950

18. Linn L: Basic principles of management in psychosomatic medicine, in Wittkower ED, Warnes H (eds): Psychosomatic Medicine Its Clinical Applications. Hagerstown, Harper & Row, 1977

19. Friedman M, Rosenman RH: Association of specific overt behavior pattern with blood and cardiovascular findings. JAMA 169:1286, 1959

20. Engel GL, Schmale AH: Psychoanalytic theory of somatic disorder: Conversion, specificity, and the disease onset situation. J Am Psychoanal Assoc 15:344−365, 1967

21. Holmes TH, Rahe RH: The social readjustment scale. J Psychosom Res 11:213, 1967

22. Masters WH, Johnson VE: Human Sexual Inadequacy. Boston, Little Brown & Co, 1970

23. Parkes CM, Benjamin B, Fitzgerald RG: Broken heart: A statistical study of increased mortality among widowers. Br Med J 1:740−743, 1969

24. Marty P, de M'Uzan M: La pensee operatoire. Rev Franc Psychoanal 27:suppl, 1963

25. Sifneos P: The prevalence of 'alexithymic' characteristics in psychosomatic patients. Psychother Psychosom 22:255−262, 1973

26. Nemiah JC: Alexithymia: Theoretical considerations. Psychother Psychosom 28:199−206, 1977

27. Hoppe K: Chronic reactive aggression in survivors of severe persecution. Comp Psychiatr 12:230−237, 1971

28. Lipowski ZJ: Psychosomatic medicine in the seventies: An overview. Am J Psychiatry 134:233−244, 1977
29. Wahl CW: The technique of brief psychotherapy with hospitalized psychosomatic patients. Int J Psychoanal Psychother 1:69−82, 1972
30. Schwab JJ, Kuhn CC: Psychiatric consultation, part II. Potential for therapy. JCE Psychiatry 40:23−31, 1979
31. Faguet RA, Fawzy FI, Wellisch DK, Pasnau RO (eds): Contemporary Models in Liaison Psychiatry. New York, Spectrum Publications, 1978
32. Pfefferbaum B, Pasnau RO, Jamison K, Wellisch DK: A comprehensive program of psychosocial care for mastectomy patients. Int J Psychiatry Med 8:63−72, 1977
33. Rahe RH, Ward HM, Hayes V: Brief group therapy in myocardial infarction rehabilitation: Three- to four-year follow-up of a controlled trial. Psychosom Med 41:229−242, 1979

Joel Yager
F. David Rudnick
Richard J. Metzner

8

Anorexia Nervosa: A Current Perspective and Some New Directions

For the researcher and clinician, anorexia nervosa presents a perplexing, fascinating and increasingly important syndrome for study and treatment. This syndrome demands multidisciplinary attention, spans several frames of reference and approaches in psychiatry and medicine, and is an excellent paradigm for the study of psychosomatic conditions involving as it does biological, developmental, psychological, and family issues. Several of its features are readily measurable, e.g. weight, and part of its attractiveness to psychiatric researchers is due to the ease with which physical measurements can be obtained. At the same time, the degree of pathology, both psychopathology and somatic pathology, is often quite severe, even life threatening. The seriousness of the illness, and its not insignificant degree of reported mortality in various series, commands the serious respect and attention of the clinician. The fact that anorexia nervosa is still being approached from so many conceptual points of view reflects our ignorance. This chapter will review some of the major clinical features of this syndrome, the major current hypotheses regarding pathogenesis and treatment, and will briefly describe a group therapy project and a television body-image confrontation project, both of which have been initiated at UCLA.

DESCRIPTION

Although cases typical of anorexia nervosa have been reported in the literature for hundreds of years;[1,2] it was not until the 1870s that Gull[3] in England and Lasegue[4] in France independently described the syndrome now known as anorexia nervosa. Although thought to be relatively rare, with an incidence of .4 to 1.6 cases per hundred thousand,[5] more recent surveys in susceptible populations have revealed a higher incidence, in the order of 1 to 200 adolescent school girls.[6] The disease is seen most frequently in women, with a ratio of only about 5 percent to 10 percent of reported cases being men,[7,8] and may have an affinity for the middle and upper middle classes. Series of cases have been reported from most Western countries, and one series of which the authors are aware has been reported from India.[9] The age of onset is most frequently in early and middle adolescence, with most cases occurring between the ages of 10 to early 20s. However, rare cases have been reported of very young children, e.g. ages 8 and 9 and younger,[10-12] and others have been reported with the onset of symptoms in the 30s and even later.[10-15] Symptoms include psychological, physical, and family problems.

Psychological Problems

In every case, anorexia nervosa presents with a determination of the patient to be thin. This is often coupled with extreme anxiety or virtually a phobia about being fat or gaining weight, and is coupled with distorted concepts about body image, attractiveness, and desirable weight.[16-18] Not infrequently, one of the earliest signs is food preoccupation with the development of culturally unusual diets, e.g. vegetarian, total elimination of certain carbohydrate-containing foods, etc., before an actual weight reduction phase begins. Voluntary restriction of the diet is often coupled with bizarre food habits. Food preoccupation occurs frequently, with obsessional thoughts concerning food and rituals around eating. In the early phases patients usually deny that anything is wrong and claim good spirits and high energy, but later on they often admit to having serious eating problems with fears of gaining weight and inability to eat. Severe and pervasive depression may then occur.[19] Food related rituals can involve food preparation, taking hours to eat meals, and eating only carefully measured quantities. In some patients rituals and compulsions extend to nonfood areas of life. Some may shoplift in bizarre fashion, e.g. only diet foods, and others may eat only from garbage cans. Some vomit repeatedly every time they eat, and some abuse laxatives or enemas in attempts to further reduce their weight. The distortion of body image can be severe, and emaciated skeleton-like creatures may interpret the slightest bulges in their abdomens as fat that demands further dieting.

The proprioception of hunger and satiety appears to be disturbed in many patients.[20] Although many patients claim that they feel hunger pangs (and, for them the term anorexia may well be a misnomer), they deliberately thwart their sensation of hunger by willfully not eating. Others, though, claim to feel reduced or absent sensation of hunger or may not be able to accurately interpret their sensations. Some feel sated after eating very small amounts of food and experience a variety of abdominal symptoms including bloating and discomfort.

A number of patients practice self-induced vomiting, often preceded by binge eating. Although in some patients this may occur relatively infrequently, e.g. several times a week, in others it may take on a major role, consuming many hours in the patient's day.[21] One of our binging vomiters, not untypical, would engage in three to four nightly binges and force herself to vomit 50 to 60 times per night, this pattern occurring for a period of years.

A considerable percentage of patients, perhaps 30 percent to 40 percent, have behavioral hyperactivity. It has recently been pointed out that hyperactivity may be one of the earliest symptoms of anorexia nervosa, prior to any weight loss.[22] Hyperactivity may take the form of exercise compulsions that lead the patient to relentlessly jog, swim, bicycle, run up and down flights of stairs, and keep active in a seemingly inexhaustible manner. Emaciated patients often continue their hyperactivity to the point of collapse. The hyperactivity may continue throughout the low weight phase, and may be one of the last symptoms to remit, after all the others have abated.

When patients are cachectic their cognitive functions are often impaired. Thinking is often "fuzzy" and may appear to be disordered; the ability to concentrate is impaired and mild signs of organicity may be seen.[10,23]

Although obsessionality is common, it is not ubiquitous. Some patients demonstrate lability of affect, histrionic, impulsive, and self-destructive behaviors.[13] Bruch has described a pervasive sense of ineffectiveness in these patients extending to all areas of life in addition to those concerning feeding.[16] Reports of suicide in a few percent of patients occur in a number of series.[10,13]

Physical Problems

A variety of physical symptoms have been associated with anorexia nervosa, most but not all of which appear to be secondary to weight loss.[24] The first symptom is a drastic weight loss. Some authorities suggest that weight loss of about 25 percent should be seen before the diagnosis is made, with suitable exceptions made in the case of still-growing adolescent girls. However, most clinicians familiar with this syndrome have seen patients with less weight loss who, nevertheless, for all intents and purposes are classic anorectics.

Amenorrhea in women in virtually universal. For the majority this occurs after the onset of menarche. In a sizable number, between about 10 percent to 20 percent, the amenorrhea precedes weight loss, and in a large percentage the amenorrhea and weight loss begin concurrently so that amenorrhea cannot be easily interpreted solely as a consequence of weight loss.[10] This observation has received considerable attention in current discussions of pathogenesis.

With severe weight loss, a large number of other physical signs and laboratory findings are recorded. These include lanugo, bradycardia, hyperkeratosis, and cold intolerance with acrocyanosis. Laboratory abnormalities include leukopenia, lymphocytosis, normochromic anemia, hypercholesterolemia, and hypercarotenemia.[24,25] In spite of the hematologic abnormalities, there is no known increase in susceptibility to infection. Except under conditions of extreme dehydration electrolytes are normal and the kidneys are spared.[26] Abnormalities in gastric emptying may be found that persist for a short period of time following weight gain.[26] The EEG is almost always normal.[27]

A variety of endocrinological abnormalities have been reported, but the large majority of them revert to normal with weight gain. These include reported abnormal elevations in cortisol levels, the presence of rT3 (an abnormal T3 variant),[28] and abnormal secretion of growth hormone.[21] Most intriguing, abnormalities in gonadotropic hormone secretion, i.e. in the regulation of LH and FSH secretion, do not appear to be solely weight related.[29,30]

Family

We note family symptoms separately because in virtually every case there are indications of significant upsets in the family at the time of the initial presentation.[31-34] Very often a worried or frantic parent is the first one to contact the physician with concern that the child may starve to death. Family issues often involve parental control and domination versus independence of thought and action in the younger adolescent. Physical separation from the home and family is often a major issue in the older adolescent and in patients in their early 20s, and ambivalent feelings and behaviors regarding separation, control, and involvement are often seen in patient and parents.

Diagnosis

The diagnosis of anorexia nervosa is usually easy to make in the full blown case. Conditions that are at times superficially similar, e.g., endocrinopathies such as pituitary or adrenal insufficiency and hyperthyroidism, are relatively easy to rule out. Anorexia-like syndromes have rarely been reported with brain lesions.[35] The subclassification of anorectic syndromes though, remains subject to debate. Some authors have differentiated primary anorexia from secondary anorexia,[18] the latter referring to other psychiatric disorders in which appetite disturbance and severe weight loss are a component. These include major affective disorders (with anorexia and weight loss) and schizophrenias which may include delusions concerning food. A variety of classifications have been suggested based on personality and defenses,[10,36] the presence of bulemia[21] and other clinical differentiating points but at present, none is universally accepted.

Conceivably, the variety of clinical manifestations may simply reflect diverse stress and coping responses to a single as yet undefined core pathological process as it is grappled with by individuals with a spectrum of cognitive styles and physiological/temperamental differences. Perhaps the concept of "anorexia spectrum disorder" may be proper. Subclinical anorexoid problems are commonly seen.

COURSE

Whether or not typical childhood antecedents exist for anorexia nervosa is open to question. Many of the children are described premorbidly as good, obedient, talented, and excellent students. Others are described as fussy eaters, temperamental, constricted, and immature.[8,10,16] A significant number, in the range of 40 percent, may be obese prior to onset,[10] and for many adolescents the onset of anorexia is heralded by the beginning of a weight reduction diet that the patient, family, and friends would all agree was indicated. However, once the diet has started and the desired amount of weight is lost, those who develop anorexia keep on dieting in spite of the increasingly anxious protests of their families.

The patient may feel exceptionally virtuous for being able to exert such self-control and willpower over the demands of the flesh. The diet and the attendant exercise appear to achieve a will of their own, not to be interfered with, as if an auto-intoxication or auto-addiction to the process or products of dieting and exercise occurs that becomes, literally, self-feeding.

Very often the precipitating event that seems to trigger the anorectic episode appears on reflection to be common to the viscissitudes of adolescent life, involving perceived rejections by friends, boy- or girl-friends, failing grades, leaving home for the first time, and the myriad of other ordinary life events of the contemporary adolescent.[10,16,37] The magnitude of the insults do not appear to be sufficiently traumatic to explain the degree of subsequent pathology.

Once the syndrome has begun, in spite of the fact that weight loss may be ⅓ to even ½ of body weight, one-half to two-thirds of the patients will regain their normal weight within a period of one to two years. However, a certain number will have repeated episodes of weight loss, and some will never regain their weight. In several series approximately 50 percent will have significant residual psychopathology,[10,16,38-40] about a third will have significant residual physical symptoms as well, and about 10 percent may be repeatedly rehospitalized. In various series, between 3 percent and 15 percent of patients die, both of malnutrition and of suicide secondary to the pervasive serious depression in chronic cases.

A number of variables have been cited that correlate with prognosis. Those that correlate with good prognosis include early age of onset, i.e. before the age of 16,[36,38,39,41,42] or onset before or within a very short time of menarche, again pointing to a young age.

Poor prognosis has been associated with older age of onset, a course of more than 7 years, a long delay of 1 to 1.5 years before seeking treatment, a very thin or very fat premorbid state,[38,39] marked personality disturbance,[38,39,41] effortless vomiting,[10] bulemia and vomiting,[10,38,41] marked parental neuroticism,[43] multiple previous treatment failures,[38,41] and severe depression.[10,38,42] While the amount of weight lost from original body weight has been related to poor prognosis in some studies,[38,39,41] others have found the amount of weight loss not to correlate with prognosis.[10]

Why earlier age of onset should be associated with good prognosis in this syndrome remains a question. The fact that this occurs even with relatively minimal treatment makes it unlikely that this finding is due to treatment effects. This situation contrasts with that in schizophrenia where, for example, earlier onset in adolescence ordinarily predicts a more malignant course. However, for certain other psychiatric symptoms, e.g. enuresis or encopresis—i.e. symptoms associated with immaturity—later onset often signifies more serious pathology.

THEORIES OF ETIOLOGY AND PATHOGENESIS

Hypotheses currently being explored relate to virtually every level of biopsychosocial organization, and these will be described in ascending order.

Genetics and Family Incidence

The genetic study of anorexia nervosa has thus far been limited. A number of cases of identical twins concordant for anorexia nervosa have been reported, but some cases of discordant identical twins have also been reported.[44-47] Some estimate prevalence of this disorder among sisters of patients to be about 6 percent to 10 percent[39,48,49] but others report lower family incidence. Among our own patients a large number have older and younger sisters with full-blown or forme-fruste anorectic syndromes. The family prevalence data, scanty as it is, cannot rule out a possible genetically mediated vulnerability. A high incidence of affective disorder[50] and of manic-depressive psychosis[49] has also been reported in the families of anoretic patients.

Another intriguing genetic finding is the possible association of anorexia nervosa with Turner's syndrome (X O karyotype). Although there is some controversy as to whether the reported number of cases in fact exceeds the number that would be expected by a chance association of these two syndromes,[51] some authors feel that the number of patients with both Turner's syndrome and anorexia is large enough to rule out chance.[52] It may be that these patients constitute a varient or subgroup of anorectic patients. It's also possible that the anorexia nervosa syndrome includes a spectrum of disorders that may be genetically heterogeneous. Definitive studies though, remain to be done.

Neurobiological Issues

A large number of neurobiological hypotheses have been advanced. One of the more interesting involves the possible pathogenetic role of hypothalamic vulnerability.[53-55] The findings that amenorrhea often precedes or coincides with weight loss and that normal cyclical release of gonadotropin may remain impaired in some patients even after weight gain point to possible weight independent abnormalities in the neuroendocrine axis. Studies using hypothalamic releasing factors have demonstrated that function of the pituitary gland per se is relatively intact,[56] suggesting abnormalities at a higher level, i.e. hypothalamus. It has been found that the secretion of LH in the thin anorectic resembles the immature secretion pattern of prepubertal girls.[57] Katz and coworkers have demonstrated that the abnormalities in the patterns of LH secretion remain even following weight gain in patients who still remain symptomatic in other ways.[58] Only those patients who both gain weight and who are otherwise symptom free have a normal LH secretion pattern.

A related hypothesis suggests that many of the features of anorexia nervosa can be accounted for by hypothalamic sensitivity to estrogen.[59] If the hypothalamus were flooded with estrogens at the start of puberty, decrease in appetite and other related symptoms might appear. A number of clinicians have reported the onset of anorectic syndromes in the context of patients starting the use of oral contraceptives.[60] We have seen that association in two patients. Whether such an association reflects primarily physiological or psychological effects of taking contraceptives is unknown.

Not surprising, possible mediating roles for brain amines have been proposed.[61,62] Abnormalities in dopamine receptor sensitivity or feedback control mechanisms have been suggested, based on the fact that such abnormalities could account for anorexia, weight loss, hyperactivity, amenorrhea, decreased libido, and other symptoms.[60] Redmond and coworkers have suggested that hyperactivity of postsynaptic noradrenergic receptors in the adrenergic satiety mechanism might be associated with pathological satiation in humans, consistent with their findings that alpha-adrenergic blocking agents can increase eating in anorexia.[63] (This is also consistent with the long recognized fact that weight gain may be associated with the use of phenothiazines, which have alpha-adrenergic blockade properties.) The behavioral similarities between anorexia nervosa and amphetaminized animals bears note, with respect to diminished appetite, weight loss, and stereotyped behavior.[64] Nevertheless, in spite of the implication of dopaminergic and alpha-adrenergic mediation, phenothiazines and butyrophenones are not specifics in the treatment of anorexia nervosa. Small peptides have also been implicated as possibly playing a role in pathogenesis.[65] The location of alpha- and beta-adrenergic mechanisms in the hypothalamic feeding areas has been demonstrated, and "eating centers" in the lateral hypothalamus and "satiety centers" in the ventromedial hypothalamus have been known for some time. It would not be surprising to learn that they are somehow involved in the expression of anorexia nervosa. Redmond et al. have also implicated the locus coeruleus in the mechanisms of satiety.[66]

The question of brain abnormalities has been raised, at least for some anorectic patients with bulemic syndromes. Rau and Green have reported soft EEG abnormalities in the right temporo-parietal region in a series of bulemic patients (only some of whom ever had anorectic syndromes), and have further reported that some of these patients responded positively to phenytoin.[67] Some, but not all, of these patients were anorectic. However, other investigators have not found anorectic bulemics to respond to phenytoin.[68]

Finally, a number of cases have been reported where patients with brain lesions, primarily tumors, have had associated anorexia-like syndromes. However, in virtually every case there are concurrent neurological findings or severe headaches that pointed to something other than garden variety anorexia nervosa.[35]

Psychodynamics

A number of psychodynamic theories have been offered to explain anorexia nervosa.[16,17,30,69-71] Unfortunately, most are based on observations made during the acute phase of the syndrome, and it is hard to separate secondary regressive consequences from primary pathogenic features. Bruch has stressed that starvation can have many meanings for the young adolescent girl.[16] For someone who feels generally ineffective and unable to achieve the perfection of the ego ideal, dieting and starvation offer methods for an exercise of willpower, asceticism, control over evil carnal impulses, self-punishment, expiation of guilt, and a chance to be either inconspicuous (i.e. frail and waif-like) or conspicuous.

The psycho-social regression has been viewed as a way of escaping from the developmental tasks of adolescence such as dealing with budding sexuality, developing heterosexual relationships, and the process of separation from the family. Children who have previously been "the perfect child" can find an acceptable form of rebellion not by acting out, but by getting sick, as a form of protest against their being oversocialized and having too many of the family's expectations projected onto them. At present no one psychodynamic theory of pathogenesis can adequately explain the variety of patients and families seen. Conceivably, the variety of psychological explanations may reflect the final common pathway nature of the diverse anorectic syndromes. Or, these psychological elements may result from rationalizations concocted by patients and their families following the onset of symptoms, developed in their attempts to understand these mysterious processes. As such they may be secondary elaborations. Many children and families with dynamics apparently similar to those described premorbidly for anorexia nervosa do not succumb, and the specific vulnerability of the susceptible person remains unexplained.

Family Theories

The interplay of the family with the sick adolescent has been thought to contribute to the pathogenesis of this disorder. Minuchin and others have stressed the transactions of families of anorectics around eating and have suggested that the patient's problems become a distraction for the family, so that the parents pay less attention to their own interpersonal difficulties at the patient's expense.[32,72] However, a starving child will generate considerable concern and overinvolvement in well-meaning parents, and this reaction is not specific for parents of anorectics.[32] A large variety of different parental attitudes and personality traits have been described, and while some have been called characteristic, no pathognomic types of family configurations have been reported.[10,43,49,73]

Once again, the description of abnormalities consequent to the illness rather than preceding it make it difficult to assign pathogenic influence to this factor in the absence of more compelling evidence.

Social and Cultural Factors

The observation that anorexia nervosa occurs largely in middle and upper-middle class patients has suggested that social factors contribute to the pathogenesis. Indeed, waves of dieting and vomiting as a method of weight control may be found in almost epidemic degrees in certain high schools and colleges.[6] Thinness, fashion model figures, and dieting are all highly valued in contemporary society, and the powers of peer pressure and the media on vulnerable adolescents must be further explored. An association with social class raises several questions, but does not necessarily point to psychogenic causation. For example, arteriosclerotic disease and peptic ulcer disease have been associated with certain social classes or groups at certain times, yet social and psychological issues per se may contribute to their appearance only to a limited extent.

TREATMENT AND PROGNOSIS

Before definite statements can be made about the efficacy of any treatment, the natural history of the syndrome must be understood. We must heed Russell's caveat that claims about treatments for anorectics may be premature unless we know the course of patients followed for a long enough period of time, e.g. at least 4 to 5 years, who have had nonspecific treatment.[74]

One of the interesting features of these syndromes is the fact that spontaneous remission, or improvement with only minimal professional help, is seen not infrequently.[42] We have met a number of women who have reported to us, after the fact, that during adolescence they suffered from anorexia nervosa with all the classic features, and after one to two years improved remarkably in their psychological, physical, and social functioning with only minimal intervention by their family physicians together with the usual attempts at persuasive coercion by their families.

Hospitalization

There is agreement that for cases with very marked weight loss, hospitalization may be necessary to help the patient regain weight. Hospitalization may be accomplished in medical, pediatric, or psychiatric units, and the choice would seem to be determined by the availability of professional staff comfortable in dealing with such patients in a given setting.[75] The purpose of weight gain, in addition to reducing the threat to life, is to improve cognitive functioning to the point where greater psychological participation of the patient may be possible. Bruch, among others, feels that the cognitive functions of severely malnourished anorectic patients may be so impaired as to preclude their profitable participation in psychotherapy.[23] Weight gain in hospital is usually accomplished by means of gentle supportive coaxing with positive incentives played against specified weight gain, and often such programs are of at least short term benefit.[74]

In severe cases where patients stubbornly refuse to gain weight, and where physical well-being is threatened, more controlling methods such as tube-feeling may be instituted. In some extreme cases hyperalimentation has been used, although some deaths have been reported as a complication of this procedure.[26] In general, it is best to avoid a contest of wills between the staff and the patient, and to allow the patient the dignity of maximum choice in participation within the context of a weight gain program. It is common, regardless of the method of treatment in hospital, to have some loss of weight following discharge, and a certain percentage of patients will require repeat hospitalization.

Behavioral Therapies

A number of programs have described successful weight gain programs for anorectics using detailed contingency schedules.[76-78] Ordinarily a certain amount of weight must be gained for the patient to be permitted specified desired privileges, such as phones, visitors, and unrestricted physical activity. Informational feedback regarding weight and intake may be essential to render reinforcement effective.[78] However, one recent multicenter study with randomized controls showed behavior therapy not to be more effective than the comparison treatments of ward milieus without behavioral programs.[79] This may reflect that a variety of subtle reinforcements (e.g. approval, demand characteristics, and expectations) inevitably exist in treatment settings and that the detailed behavioral programs don't add much to these powerful influences. Bruch has stressed that the short-term weight gains with behavioral intervention may result in negative long-term effects with respect to the patient's ultimate cooperation with treatment.[80]

Psychodynamic Therapy

There is general agreement that supportive, reality oriented psychotherapy may benefit patients with this syndrome.[16,17] Although classic psychoanalytic therapy appears to be contraindicated, a noncritical collaborative enterprise between a psychotherapist and the patient may be quite useful. Issues that warrant exploration include the patient's fears of ineffectiveness and inadequacy, the pursuit of perfection, the turmoils of adolescent development including sexuality, and the patient's need for control, among others. Even with such therapy though, residual psychiatric problems in about half the patients remain considerable.[16,38,40]

Family Therapy

The importance of the family in the therapy of anorexia nervosa has been recognized by a number of writers. Some have described active family therapies where family members are used as collaborative agents for helping to establish behavioral weight gain programs in the home.[81,82] Included, too, are structural family therapy approaches whereby, in part, active intervention is aimed at refocusing some of the family's concern away from the symptoms of the child to other issues in the family.[72,82,83] Minuchin et al.[71] cite the relatively good outcome of their patients treated by methods of structural family therapy. However, their patients are generally of the younger and therefore better prognosis group, making it difficult to fully assess the comparative benefits of this approach.

Medications

Although a number of psychopharmacological agents have been used in the treatment of anorexia nervosa, at present no one drug appears to hold the answer. Cyproheptadine, an antihistaminic and antiserotonergic agent, has been associated with greater weight gain than placebo in double-blind studies.[84] It may serve in part as an appetite stimulant. Nevertheless, the results are modest, and in our experience some patients are reluctant to take the medication for the very reason that it stimulates the appetite.

Tricyclic antidepressants may be useful for some patients.[85-87] It has been suggested for theoretical reasons that amitryptiline may be more useful than imipramine because of its predominantly serotonin rather than norepinephrine reuptake blockade properties.[87] However, no careful studies have been done using antidepressants and results in the hands of many clinicians have been variable.

Phenothiazines and butyrophenones have been used for some patients. Weight gain may be rapid with patients on phenothiazines,[10] yet many patients often lose the weight just as rapidly once the medication is discontinued. In some patients, these medications may be useful in reducing anxiety and compulsions, but again the results are variable.

Lithium has been used in some patients, but especially in patients who vomit and who use diuretics its use is not indicated.[88]

Phenytoin has been reported to be of use in some patients with a binge-vomiting syndrome, especially with patients who have soft EEG abnormalities. However, the percentage of patients who will respond in this way is small, and apparently the relationship between patients who benefit and who have EEG abnormalities, is not precise.[67,68]

Other somatic therapies such as insulin (for appetite stimulation) and electroconvulsive therapy have been employed but are not in vogue, and demonstrate no particular advantage.[10]

Group Therapies

Over the last few years a number of self-help groups have emerged across the country (e.g., Anorexia Aid Society), but their contribution to the overall problem has not yet been assessed. Therapy groups for anorexic patients are being conducted in several centers (e.g., NIMH, Cleveland Clinics), but these have not yet been described in the professional literature.

A PILOT GROUP PROJECT

A group psychotherapy program for anorectic patients has been conducted at UCLA's Neuropsychiatric Institute by two of the authors (JY, FDR), and this section will briefly describe some features of that program.

An initial group, now terminated, ran weekly for one and a half years and at its largest, involved nine patients. The youngest patient was 18 and the oldest 34. Most patients were in their mid-20s, and all were women. One was married, one divorced, and the remainder were single. All but one patient had already left the parental home. The duration of their eating problems ranged from 1 to about 15 years, averaging 4 to 5 years. The age of onset in this group tended to be late, i.e. over 16 for all but one of the patients. Five patients had problems with thinness, of whom two were hyperactive; three who were previously thin now had binge-vomiting as their major problem; one, previously thin, had residual problems of personality structure. At some time during the group virtually every patient was in another form of treatment besides group therapy, such as individual or family therapy, and some were receiving medications. Therefore, changes in status cannot clearly be attributed to influences of the group.

From our point of view the purpose of the group was heuristic. We proposed to use the group method as a vehicle for seeing the varieties of the anorexia syndrome, having the patients confirm or disconfirm hypotheses and observations presented in the literature, and for suggesting new directions for investigation through their interactions. Our methods were open-ended, based primarily on dynamic group and combined insight-oriented and supportive approaches with occasional topic-oriented discussions, e.g. in the formulation of problem lists. We placed no restrictions on, and indeed encouraged, the development of outside relationships.

From the patients' point of view, the benefits of the group consisted of their meeting people with similar problems, sharing experiences, feeling less "freaky", and developing friendships. They felt that the group leaders and other patients were among the few people that they had met who could really understand their problems, and they found this to be a source of comfort. However, the group also imposed its own problems on them. These included having to be labeled as a certain type of patient, and concentrating and focusing on their symptoms and illness. For some, the task of having to look in a nonescapable way at some of their common dynamics and "games" was more than they could easily bear. The overt expression of anger was very threatening to several in the group.

Our summary impression is that dynamic group psychotherapy can offer a useful adjunctive experience to patients with chronic anorexia, but it is not in and of itself either an adequate or sufficient treatment.

VIDEO TAPE BODY IMAGE CONFRONTATION

Since distortion of the body image is central and significant in anorexia nervosa, refined techniques to explore this feature may yield important pathogenic and therapeutic information. Thus far a variety of static visual techniques, e.g. estimations of body width and body shadows, have been used by several investigators.[89-92] To our knowledge video tape has not been used in this fashion. One case report describes the use of audio-visual feedback over an extended period of time as one component in the treatment of an anorectic patient.[93]

Thus far we have used television recording and playback to explore body-image distortion in five anorectic patients. The technique consists of a 15 to 20 minute video tape interview during which the patient stands and moves in a bikini bathing suit. During this interview, a psychiatrist questions the patient about her perceptions and sentiments about each individual part of her body, and her body as a whole. The cameras record total and part body pictures from the front, side, back, and from a variety of angles. Approximately one week later the patient is brought back to the television studio to watch the initial video tape. During the playback the psychiatrist discusses the patient's impressions of the initial session with her, and the playback is itself recorded.

With this small series, only preliminary statements can be made. We have thus far seen three distinct types of reactions to video tape playback. The first can be labeled *concept-percept dissonance*. In this situation the patient's internal conception of her body (usually that she is too heavy) is at variance with how she perceives it on television. The response is astonishment, disgust, and emotionality. One patient who most dramatically demonstrated this reaction had, on a 17-month follow-up, a remarkable weight gain after having been chronically thin for several years. She subsequently attributed her internal change in motivation to gain weight, at least in part, to the powerful impact the initial video playback had made upon her.

The second reaction is *concept-percept congruence*. In this situation, the patient claims an accurate self-concept, i.e. that of being very thin and emaciated. Here, the playback of the thin body causes no great surprise. The patient may have either the determination to remain thin, as she views herself both internally and on the screen, or she may voice the desire to gain weight, appreciating her actual situation yet unable to overcome the internal resistances.

The third reaction is *concept-percept confusion*. In this situation a patient may claim that she is unable to interpret or to judge either her internal body image or the one that she sees on the screen. That is, she lacks an adequate sense of what she should look like, what is "good and right", and what she wants for herself. This state of confusion may resolve and be replaced with a more realistic and definable body concept later in the patient's course.

Although we have not studied this method as a treatment technique, the weight gain in the patient who experienced the most dramatic reaction to video tape confrontation suggests that in selected patients, e.g. those with *concept-percept dissonance*, the repeated use of video tape playback may be a powerful adjunctive treatment technique.

CONCLUSION

Anorexia nervosa remains an enigmatic syndrome. The diversity of clinical features suggests the possibility of as yet ill defined subtypes, and the many current pathogenic hypotheses and treatment approaches attest to our embryonic state of knowledge.

Most workers clearly recognize that the problems surrounding weight are but one small component of these complex syndromes that involve biological, psychological, family and social issues. Further attention to basic research and clinical practice aspects are warranted by virtue of the seriousness of these disorders and their apparently increasing prevalence in the population.

REFERENCES

1. Shafii M: A precedent for modern psychotherapeutic techniques: One thousand years ago. Am J Psychiatry 128:1581−1584, 1972
2. Morton R: Phthisiologia—or a Treatise on Consumption. London, Smith, 1689
3. Gull WW: Anorexia nervosa (apepsia hysterica, anorexia hysterica). Transactions of the Clinical Society of London 7:22−28, 1874

4. Lasèque C: De l'anorexie hystérique. Archives Générales de Médecine 1:385–403, 1873
5. Kendell RE, Hall D, Hailey A, et al: The epidemiology of anorexia nervosa. Psychol Med 3:200–203, 1973
6. Crisp AH, Palmer RL, Kalucy RS: How common is anorexia nervosa? A prevelance study. Br J Psychiatry 128:549–554, 1976
7. Bruch H: Anorexia nervosa in the male. Psychosom Med 33:31–47, 1971
8. Halmi KA: Anorexia nervosa: Demographic and clinical features of 94 cases. Psychosom Med 36:18–26, 1974
9. Rao NVS Surya Prakash: Adjustment reactions of childhood. Child Psychiatry Quarterly (Hyderbad) 10:8–26, 1977
10. Dally P: Anorexia Nervosa. London, Wm Heineman Ltd, 1969
11. Shafii M, Salguero C, Finch SM: Anorexia a deux: Psychopathology and treatment of anorexia nervosa in latency age siblings. J Am Acad Child Psychiatry 14:617–632, 1975
12. Rank B, Putnam MC, Rochlin G: The significance of the "emotional climate" in early feeding disturbance. Psychosom Med 10:279–283, 1948
13. Seidensticher JF, Tzagournis M: Anorexia nervosa—clinical features and long term follow up. J Chronic Dis 21:361–367, 1968
14. Ryle JA: Anorexia Nervosa: The Natural History of Disease. London, Oxford University Press, 1948, pp 118–129
15. Kellett JM, Trimble M, Thorley AP: Anorexia nervosa after the menopause. Brit J Psychiatry 128:555–558, 1976
16. Bruch H: Eating Disorders. New York, Basic Books, 1973, pp 211–305
17. Crisp AH: Clinical and therapeutic aspects of anorexia nervosa—a study of 30 cases. J Psychosomatic Res 9:67–78, 1965
18. King A: Primary and secondary anorexia nervosa syndromes. Brit J Psychiatry 109:470–479, 1963
19. Casper RC, Davis JM: On the course of anorexia nervosa. Am J Psychiatry 134:974–978, 1977
20. Garfinkel PE: Perception of hunger and satiety in anorexia nervosa. Psychol Med 4:309–315, 1974
21. Beumont P, George G, Smart D: Dieters and vomiters and purgers in anorexia nervosa. Psychol Med 6:617–622, 1976
22. Kron L, Katz JL, Gorzynski G, et al: Hyperactivity in anorexia nervosa: A fundamental clinical feature. Compr Psychiatry 19:433–440, 1978
23. Bruch H: The Golden Cage. Cambridge, Mass., Harvard University Press, 1978
24. Halmi KA: Anorexia nervosa: Recent investigations. Ann Rev Med 29:137–148, 1978
25. Warren MP, VandeWie RL: Clinical and metabolic features of anorexia nervosa. Am J Obstetrics and Gynecology 117:435–449, 1973
26. Silverman J: Medical complications of anorexia nervosa. Panel presentation at American Psychiatric Association 131st Meeting. Atlanta, Georgia, 1978
27. Anderson AE: Medical complications of anorexia nervosa. Panel presentation at American Psychiatric Association 131st Meeting. Atlanta, Georgia, 1978

28. Boyar RM, Hellman LD, Roffwarg H, et al: Cortisol secretion and metabolism in anorexia nervosa. New Eng J Med 296:190–193, 1977

29. Vigersky RA, Loriaux DL, Anderson AE, et al: Delayed pituitary hormone response to LRF and TRF in patients with anorexia nervosa and with secondary amenorrhea associated with simple weight loss. J Clin End and Metab 43:893–900, 1976

30. Katz JL, Boyar R, Roffwarg H, et al: Weight and circadian luteinizing hormone secretory pattern in anorexia nervosa. Psychosom Med 40:549–567, 1978

31. Dally P: Anorexia nervosa: Do we need a scapegoat? Proceedings Royal Society of Med 70:470–474, 1977

32. Minuchin S, Baker L, Rosman BL, et al: A conceptual model of psychosomatic illness in children: Family organization and family therapy. Arch Gen Psychiatry 32:1031–1038, 1975

33. Conrad DE: A starving family: An interactional view of anorexia nervosa. Bull Menninger Clin 41:487–495, 1977

34. Wold P: Family structure in three cases of anorexia nervosa: The role of the father. Am J Psychiatry 130:1394–1397, 1973

35. Lundberg PO, Walinder J: Anorexia nervosa and signs of brain damage. Int J Neuropsychiatry 1:165–173, 1967

36. Lesser LI, Ashenden BJ, Delruskey M, et al: Anorexia nervosa in children. Am J Orthopsychiatry 30:572–580, 1960

37. Beumont PJV, Abraham SF, Argall WJ, et al: The onset of anorexia nervosa. Austr New Z J Psychiatry 12:145–149, 1978

38. Hsu LKG, Crisp AH, Harding B: Outcome in anorexia nervosa. Lancet 1:61–65, 1979

39. Morgan HG, Russell GFM: Value of family background and clinical features as predictors of long term outcome in anorexia nervosa: Four year follow-up of 41 patients. Psychological Medicine 5:355–371, 1975

40. Kay DWK, Leigh D: The natural history, treatment and prognosis of anorexia nervosa based on a study of 38 patients. J Mental Science 100:411–431, 1954

41. Halmi K, Brodland G, Lonely J: Prognosis in anorexia nervosa. Ann Int Med 78:907–909, 1973

42. Goetz PL, Succop RA, Reinhart JB, et al: Anorexia nervosa in children: A follow-up study. Amer J Orthopsychiat 47:597–603, 1977

43. Crisp AH, Harding B, McGuiness B: Anorexia nervosa. Psychoneurotic characteristics of patients: Relationship to prognosis. J Psychosomatic Research 18:167–173, 1974

44. Halmi KA, Brodland G: Monozygotic twins: Concordant and discordant for anorexia nervosa. Psychological Medicine 3:521–524, 1973

45. Neki JS, Mohan D, Sood RK: Anorexia nervosa in a monozygotic twin pair. J Indian Med Assoc (Calcutta) 68:98–100, 1977

46. Wiener JM: Identical male twins discordant for anorexia nervosa: A case study. J Child Psychiatry 15:523–534, 1976

47. Bemis KM: Current approaches to the etiology and treatment of anorexia nervosa. Psychol Bull 85:593–617, 1978

48. Theander S: Anorexia nervosa. Acta Psychiatrica Scandinavica Suppl 214:38−51, 1970
49. Kalucy RS, Crisp AH, Harding B: A study of 56 families with anorexia nervosa. Br J Med Psychol 50:381−395, 1977
50. Cantwell DP, Sturzenberger S, Burroughs J, et al: Anorexia nervosa: An affective disorder? Arch Gen Psychiatry 34:1087−1093, 1977
51. Liston EH, Shershow LW: Concurrence of anorexia nervosa and gonadal dysgenesis. Arch Gen Psychiatry 29:834−836, 1973
52. Kron L, Katz J, Gorzynski G, et al: Anorexia nervosa and gonadal dysgenesis: Further evidence of a relationship. Arch Gen Psychiatry 34:332−335, 1977
53. Russel GFM: Anorexia nervosa: Its identity as an illness and its treatment, in Price SH (ed): Modern Trends in Psychological Medicine 2. London, Butterworths, 1972, pp 131−164
54. Mecklenberg RS, Loriaux DL, Thompson RH, et al: Hypothalamic dysfunction in patients with anorexia nervosa. Medicine 53:147−159, 1974
55. Katz JL, Weiner H: A functional anterior hypothalamic defect in primary anorexia nervosa? Psychosom Med 37:103−105, 1975
56. Katz JL, Boyar RM, Roffwarg H, et al: LHRH responsiveness in anorexia nervosa: Intactness despite prepubertal circadian LH pattern. Psychosom Med 34:241−251, 1977
57. Boyar RM, Katz J, Finkelstein JW, et al: Immaturity of the 24 hour luteinizing hormone secretory pattern. New Engl J Med 291:862−865, 1974
58. Katz JL, Boyar R, Roffwarg H, et al: Weight and circadian LH secretory patterns in anorexia nervosa. Psychosom Med 40:549−567, 1978
59. Young JK: A possible neuroendocrine basis of two clinical syndromes: Anorexia nervosa and Klein-Levin syndrome. Physiol Psychology 3:322−330, 1975
60. Fries H, Nillius SJ: Dieting, anorexia nervosa and amenorrhea after oral contraceptive treatment. Acta Psychiatrica Scandinavica 49:669−679, 1973
61. Mawson AR: Anorexia nervosa and the regulation of intake: A review. Psychol Med 4:289−308, 1974
62. Barry VC, Klawans HL: On the role of dopamine in the pathophysiology of anorexia nervosa. J Neural Transmission 38:107−122, 1976
63. Redmond DE, Swann A, Heninger GR: Phenoxybenzamine in anorexia nervosa. Lancet 2:307, 1976
64. Segal DS: Personal Communication. Department of Psychiatry, UC San Diego, 1977
65. Reichelt KL, Trygstad O, Foss I, et al: Peptides in CNS control of diseases. Acta Pharmacologica et Toxicologica (Copenhagen) 41 (suppl):27, 1977
66. Redmond DE, Huang YH, Snyder Dr, et al: Hyperphagia and hyperdipsia after locus coeruleus lesions in the Stumptailed monkey. Life Sciences 20:1619−1628, 1977
67. Green RS, Rau JH: Treatment of compulsive eating disturbances with anticonvulsant medication. Am J Psychiatry 131:428−432, 1974
68. Wermuth BM, Davis KL, Hollister LE, et al: Phenytoin treatment of the binge-eating syndrome. Am J Psychiatry 134:1249−1253, 1977

69. Kaufman MR, Heiman M (eds): Evolution of Psychosomatic Concepts of Anorexia Nervosa: A Paradigm. New York, International Universities Press, 1964

70. Thoma H: Anorexia Nervosa. New York, International Universities Press, 1967

71. Palazzoli MS: Self Starvation. New York, Jason Aronson, 1978

72. Minuchin S, Rosman BL, Baker L: Psychosomatic Families: Anorexia Nervosa in Context. Cambridge, Mass., Harvard University Press, 1978

73. Halmi KA, Struss A, Goldberg SC: An investigation of weights in the parents of anorexia nervosa patients. J Nerv Ment Dis 166:358−361, 1978

74. Russell GFM: General management of anorexia nervosa and difficulties in assessing the efficacy of treatment, in Vigersky RA (ed): Anorexia Nervosa. New York, Raven Press, 1977, pp 277−289

75. Maxmen JS, Silberfarb PM, Ferrell RB: Anorexia nervosa: Practical initial management in a general hospital. JAMA 229:801−803, 1974

76. Blinder BJ, Freeman DMA, Stunkard AJ: Behavior therapy of anorexia nervosa: Effectiveness of activity as a reinforcer of weight gain. Am J Psychiatry 126:1093−1098, 1970

77. Stunkard AJ: New therapies for the eating disorders. Arch Gen Psychiatry 26:391−398, 1972

78. Agras S, Werne J: Behavior modification in anorexia nervosa research foundations, in Vigersky RA (ed): Anorexia Nervosa. New York, Raven Press, 1977, pp 291−303

79. Eckert ED, Goldberg SC, Halmi KA, et al: Behavior therapy in anorexia nervosa. Brit J Psychiatry 134:55−59, 1979

80. Bruch H: Perils of behavior modification in treatment of anorexia nervosa. JAMA 230:1419−1422, 1974

81. Barcai A: Family therapy in the treatment of anorexia nervosa. Am J Psychiatry 128:286−290, 1971

82. Rosman BL, Minuchin S, Liebman R: Family lunch session: An introduction to family therapy in anorexia nervosa. Am J Orthopsychiatry 45:846−853, 1975

83. Perlman LM, Bender SS: Operant reinforcement with structural family therapy in training anorexia nervosa. J Family Counseling 3:38−46, 1975

84. Goldberg SC, Halmi KA, Eckert ED: Cyproheptadine in anorexia nervosa. Brit J Psychiatry 134:67−70, 1979

85. Mills IH, Wilson RJ, Eden MAM, et al: Endocrine and social factors in self-starvation amenorrhea, in Robertson RF, Proudfoot AT (eds): Anorexia Nervosa and Obesity (symposium). Royal College of Physicians of Edinburgh, 1973 pp 31−43

86. Needleman HL, Waber D: Amitryptaline therapy in patients with anorexia nervosa. Lancet 2:580, 1976

87. Moore DC: Amitryptyline therapy in anorexia nervosa. Am J Psychiatry 134:1303−1304, 1977

88. Barcai A: Lithium in adult anorexia nervosa: A pilot report in two patients. Acta Psychiatrica Scandinavica 55:97−101, 1977

89. Slade PD, Russell GFM: Awareness of body dimensions in anorexia nervosa:

Cross-sectional and longitudinal studies. Psychol Med 3:188–199, 1973

90. Crisp AH, Kalucy RS: Aspects of the perceptual disorder in anorexia nervosa. Br J Med Psychol 47:349–361, 1974

91. Garner DM, Garfinkel PE, Stancer HC, et al: Body image disturbances in anorexia nervosa and obesity. Psychosom Med 38:327–336, 1976

92. Casper RC, Halmi KA, Goldberg S, et al: Disturbances in body image estimation as related to other characteristics and outcome of anorexia nervosa. Br J Psychiatry 134:60–66, 1979

93. Gottheil E, Backup CE, Cornelison FS, Jr.: Denial and self-image confrontation in a case of anorexia nervosa. J Nerv Ment Dis 148:238–250, 1969

Donald S. Hiroto
Stefanie Doyle Peters

9
Learned Helplessness: A Laboratory Model of Depression

Depression, with its debilitating and sometimes fatal consequences, is the most common of the major psychiatric disorders, and it can occur at any point in the life cycle, from infancy to old age.[1-4] Depressive disorders are extremely heterogeneous with respect to symptomatology, severity, course, and hypothesized etiological factors. Such complexity poses considerable problems for the clinical investigator, and much current research is directed towards differentiating well defined sub-types within the family of depressive disorders.

One approach to the study of psychopathology is the use of a laboratory model in which an experimentally produced phenomenon is viewed as an analogue of some naturally occurring disorder. In the area of depression, this approach is most closely associated with Seligman's learned helplessness model.[5] The term "learned helplessness" describes what happens to individuals when they learn that their responses have no effect on changing important parts of their lives. This experience of learning that outcomes are uncontrollable produces a characteristic syndrome of behavioral, cognitive, and motivational deficits. Because these deficits closely resemble certain depressive symptoms, Seligman has proposed that learned helplessness could serve as a model for reactive depression.[5-7]

Over the past decade, learned helplessness theory has generated a large number of research studies. The first portion of this chapter will review the empirical and conceptual development of the theory, from its beginnings in the field of animal learning, to its current status as a comprehensive cognitive social-learning approach to human behavior. The second part will then evaluate the appropriateness of learned helplessness as a model of depression and discuss how the model might be used to increase our understanding of the depressive disorders.

DEVELOPMENT OF LEARNED HELPLESSNESS THEORY

Research with Animals

Learned helplessness theory had its origins in an accidental, but highly fortuitous, discovery which occurred during a laboratory study of animal learning. It was found that dogs exposed to inescapable, uncontrollable shock were subsequently unable to learn simple escape responses when placed in a situation where shock was controllable. Overmier and Seligman[8] and Seligman and Maier[9] coined the term "learned helplessness" to describe this intriguing phenomenon and undertook a more systematic investigation of the effects of uncontrollability. The following summary of their early studies with animals should provide the reader with both a fuller understanding of the helplessness phenomenon and an outline of the basic experimental paradigm and triadic research design that are now characteristic of helplessness research.

The learned helplessness paradigm always involves a two-phase laboratory procedure. During the first, or training, phase, the organism is exposed to some form of uncontrollable event. Uncontrollability is defined here as a condition in which the outcomes experienced by the organism are independent of its responses. In the early animal studies, dogs were placed in hammocks and given a series of electric shocks. These shocks, while not harmful to the animals, were aversive and uncontrollable. The second phase of the procedure is designed to test for the effects of uncontrollability by placing the organism in a situation where outcomes are now contingent upon its responses. Typically, the test phase has involved placing the dog in an apparatus called a shuttle-box. This is a long, rectangular enclosure with metal rods in the floor and a shoulder-high barrier down the middle. When shock is administered through the floor on one side of the box, the animal simply has to jump over the barrier to escape.

Seligman and Maier[9] divided the animals in their study into three experimental groups. Dogs in the first (nonhelpless) group were able to terminate the shock by pressing a panel with their noses or heads. Dogs in the helpless group were yoked to those in the first group so that the shocks experienced by the two groups were identical in duration and intensity. Thus, the helpless dogs received a programmed series of shocks over which they had no control. The third group of animals constituted a naive control group and was not given any shock. This triadic research design has become a central feature of learned helplessness experiments since it enables researchers to differentiate the effects of uncontrollability from those of aversive stimuli.

When tested later in a shuttle-box, both naive dogs and dogs pretreated with controllable shock were able to learn the escape response within a few trials. However, the dogs that had experienced uncontrollable shock characteristically became passive and failed to try to escape. Even if one of these dogs did, at some point, succeed in jumping the barrier, it would typically revert to passive acceptance of the shock on later trials, suggesting that the animal failed to associate jumping with the termination of shock. Seligman[5] vividly describes the behavior of one of the helpless dogs as follows (p 22):

> This dog's first reactions to shock in the shuttle-box were much the same as those of a naive dog: it ran around frantically for about thirty seconds. But then it stopped moving; to our surprise, it lay down and quietly whined. After one minute of this we turned the shock off; the dog had failed to cross the barrier and had not escaped from shock. On the next trial, the dog did it again; at first it struggled a bit, and then, after a few seconds, it seemed to give up and to accept the shock passively. On all succeeding trials, the dog failed to escape. This is the paradigmatic learned helplessness finding.

To summarize then, learned helplessness in dogs is defined by two types of deficits: (1) failure to initiate responses (or marked retardation in responding); and (2) interference with subsequent learning that responding is effective. Further research has shown that these findings are neither isolated nor restricted to dogs. The helplessness phenomenon has been replicated by a number of studies using various species and experimental conditions (e.g., refs. 10−14).

The relative permanence or transience of helpless effects depends in part on how the uncontrollable stimulus is administered.[8,12] The effects tend to be time-limited when a series of shocks is delivered during one laboratory session. An animal that was initially helpless can be tested again several days later and learn to escape normally. However, if the same total number of shocks is administered over several days, interference with learning becomes relatively chronic: dogs can be retested in the shuttle-box weeks or months later and still fail to escape. It has also been shown that animals could develop some degree of immunization against the effects of inescapable shock if they were given experience with controllable shock prior to receiving helplessness training.[9]

The term learned helplessness refers not only to the two main deficits described earlier but also to the hypothesis about the underlying processes responsible for producing these deficits. Maier, Seligman, and Solomon proposed that helplessness effects result from learning that outcomes are not contingent on responses.[10] The organism's expectation that outcomes are uncontrollable leads to both motivational deficits, such as retarded initiation of responses, and cognitive deficits in the form of interference with later learning that responses are associated with outcomes. This postulated connection between behavioral deficits and expectations of uncontrollability forms the core of the learned helplessness hypothesis.

Research with Humans

Once the phenomenon of learned helplessness was well established in animals, researchers began to question whether parallel effects would occur when human subjects were exposed to uncontrollable events. One of the first studies to address this issue was conducted by Hiroto, using a loud unpleasant noise as the aversive stimulus.[15] The subjects were college students who were divided into three groups in keeping with the triadic research design described in the previous section. The nonhelpless group could terminate the noise by pressing a button. For the helpless group, the aversive stimulus was uncontrollable since termination of noise occurred independently of button-pressing. A third group of students was not exposed to noise during the training phase of the experiment.

The effects of helplessness training were then tested by asking all three groups of subjects to terminate noise using a hand shuttle-box. This apparatus was somewhat analogous to the animal shuttle-box in that subjects had to learn to slide a handle from one end of the box to the other in order to turn off the noise. The results of this study clearly paralleled the helplessness effects found in animals. Subjects who had been exposed to controllable noise or no noise in the first phase of the experiment learned to use the hand shuttle-box equally well. However, the helpless subjects, those previously exposed to uncontrollable noise, exhibited a number of behavioral deficits in the test phase. They took significantly longer to turn the noise off, made more errors before finding the solution, and were slower in moving the handle than subjects in either of the other two groups.

In addition, Hiroto was concerned with investigating the hypothesis that expectancy of uncontrollability was the major factor underlying helplessness effects. This hypothesis was examined in two ways. First, students were preselected for the study based on scores from the Internal-External Locus of Control Inventory.[16] This inventory presumably identifies individuals who believe that they control events in their lives (internals) versus those who believe their lives are controlled by outside forces or other persons (externals). Second, subjects' perceptions of the shuttle-box task were manipulated by the experimenter. Half the subjects were told the solution depended on skill, and half that it depended on chance.

When subjects were divided according to Locus of Control, Hiroto found that those who typically expected uncontrollability (externals) were more susceptible to the effects of inescapable noise than the internals, who tended to believe that they had personal control over their lives. The results also showed that students who were led to believe that the shuttle-box solution was based on chance factors were more helpless than students who were led to believe that the task was based on skill factors. Taken together, these findings suggest that intensification of helplessness effects is associated with other factors, either preexisting or experimentally imposed, that encourage subjects to form general expectancies of uncontrollability. Thus, Hiroto's results support the hypothesis that such expectancies are the mechanism by which the experience of uncontrollability produces helplessness deficits.

Further support for this hypothesis was provided by Hiroto and Seligman's study on the generality of helplessness effects.[17] They reasoned that if learned helplessness were a specific state mediated by environmental cues, impaired performance would occur only in situations similar to the original training. If, on the other hand, helplessness were produced by an internal state of the organism—namely, the expectancy of uncontrollabality—its effects should generalize across different stimulus and response modalities. The results of their study strongly supported the latter proposition. Students who were first exposed to inescapable loud noise, in comparison to students given escapable noise or no noise, subsequently exhibited deficits in cognitive performance when asked to solve simple anagrams. Likewise, experience with insoluble cognitive problems later produced impaired instrumental performance in learning to terminate noise using the hand shuttle-box.

There is now a substantial body of literature documenting the various conditions associated with human helplessness (e.g., refs. 18−27). Some of these findings parallel the results of studies of animal helplessness. Performance deficits appear to be more likely when the amount of exposure to uncontrollable events is increased. Conversely, prior experience with controllable outcomes provides some degree of immunization against helplessness effects in humans, just as it does in animals.

The use of human subjects has also given researchers the opportunity to explore the cognitive mediating processes involved in learned helplessness. For example, Roth and Kubal[26] and Miller and Gold[28] have demonstrated that perceived importance of the task is crucial to the development of helplessness. These studies used very similar procedures in which two groups of subjects were given the same insoluble task but different instructional sets. One group was told the task was an index of scholastic and academic achievement, while the second group was given an innocuous description which minimized the importance of the task. The findings were the same for both studies. Subjects who had received the highly important manipulation showed a significantly impaired performance in the test phase of the experiment, but those in the unimportant condition showed no impairment at all. So, the production of helplessness depends not only on the experience of uncontrollability, but also on the specific meaning that the individual attaches to the outcome in question.

The Reformulated Model of Learned Helplessness

The initial learned helplessness model postulated that the experience of uncontrollability led to expectancies of future uncontrollability which, in turn, produced deficits in motivation and cognitive abilities. However, in recent years it became apparent that this model, which originated in studies of animals, did not adequately account for all of the empirical findings concerning human helplessness. Therefore, Abramson, Seligman, and Teasdale have revised and reformulated the model in order to address themselves specifically to the cognitive processes involved in human helplessness.[29] The basic assumption underlying the reformulation is the following: "In brief, we argue that when a person finds that he is helpless, he asks why he is helpless. The causal attribution he makes then determines the generality and chronicity of his helplessness deficits as well as his later self-esteem" (p 50).

Since the reformulated model is essentially an attributional analysis, it will be helpful to provide the reader with a brief introduction to attribution theory, particularly the work of Weiner and his associates, before proceeding with our discussion of learned helplessness. Attribution research is concerned primarily with individuals' perceptions of causality.[30,31] It is guided by the assumption that humans are motivated to find reasons for the successes and failures they experience. These causal attributions are then important determinants of both affective responses to various events, and expectations about future outcomes.[32] For example, an individual who attributed success to luck would experience a positive emotional reaction but might not increase his or her expectations of future success. Failures which are attributed to personal inadequacies are likely to be especially devastating since they result in both negative affect and increased expectations of failure in the future.

The reformulated model of learned helplessness posits that the individual first perceives that responses and outcomes are independent and then makes an attribution about the cause of his or her helplessness. The causal attribution determines the person's expectancy of future uncontrollability which, in turn, determines the nature and severity of the resulting deficits. Specifically, Abramson et al. propose that the type, the chronicity, and the generality of learned helplessness effects can be understood more fully when causal attributions are categorized along the following three orthogonal dimensions: internal-external; stable-unstable; and global-specific.

Internal-External. Causal attributions can be made to factors internal to the person (such as ability or mood) or to factors which are external (such as luck or the behavior of others). This distinction between internal and external attributions led Abramson et al. to posit that there are two different types of helplessness, which they label "personal" and "universal" Personal helplessness occurs when one perceives that outcomes are not contingent on any responses in one's own repertoire but are controllable by others. Thus, a man who believed he lost his job because he was incompetent compared to his coworkers would be experiencing personal helplessness. In contrast, universal helplessness occurs when there is consensual agreement that no one could control a particular outcome. Natural disasters and terminal illness are extreme examples of circumstances in which individuals would experience universal helplessness. An important implication of the distinction between these two types of helplessness is that lowered self-esteem is believed to occur only in conjunction with personal helplessness.

Stable-Unstable. Attributions can also be analyzed along the dimension of stability. Stable attributions refer to factors like intellectual ability or physical attractiveness which are relatively invariant over time. More variable factors, such as luck or temporary fatigue, are considered to be unstable attributions. Abramson et al. suggest that deficits will tend to be chronic when individuals make stable attributions about their helplessness but relatively transient if their attributions are to unstable causes.

Global-Specific. Finally, causal attributions can be categorized as being either global or specific. Global factors are those which affect a wide range of outcomes, while specific factors are much more limited in their effects. The more global the attribution made by an individual, the more likely it is that helplessness will generalize to situations quite different from the original situation in which uncontrollability was experienced. Thus, a student who attributes her poor performance on a history exam to "being bad at history" will probably experience less impairment in other academic areas than one who attributes her failure to a more global cause like "being stupid".

Both the original and the reformulated models hold that the expectancy of uncontrollability is the critical factor underlying learned helplessness. In other words, helplessness will occur only if the perception of response-outcome independence in the present is transformed into an expectation that such independence will exist in the future. The original model, though, was vague in specifying the conditions under which this transformation would take place. The incorporation of an attributional framework enables the reformulated model to resolve this inadequacy and to make more precise predictions about the nature of the expected deficits in a given situation. However, since the reformulation is a very recent development in learned helplessness theory, it has not yet received extensive empirical testing.

LEARNED HELPLESSNESS AND DEPRESSION

The helplessness hypothesis has inspired a number of intriguing studies which have investigated the relationship of uncontrollability to such diverse phenomena as aging,[33,34] heart disease,[35,36] environmental stress,[37,38] and emotional development.[5,19,20] But the major thrust of the research has been directed towards assessing the parallels between human helplessness and depression.

Several years ago, Seligman noted the manifest similarities between helplessness deficits and depressive symptoms and suggested that learned helplessness might serve as a laboratory model for certain types of depression, particularly those labelled "reactive" or "exogenous".[5-7] Abramson, Seligman, and Teasdale,[29] in their reformulation of learned helplessness theory, present the following model of depression (p 68):

1. Depression consists of four classes of deficits: motivational, cognitive, self-esteem, and affective.
2. When highly desired outcomes are believed improbable, or highly aversive outcomes are believed probable and the individual expects that no response in his repertoire will change their likelihood, (helplessness) depression results.
3. The generality of the depressive deficits will depend on the globality of the attribution for helplessness, the chronicity of the depression deficits will depend on the stability of the attribution for helplessness, and whether self-esteem is lowered will depend on the internality of the attribution for helplessness.
4. The intensity of the deficits depends on the strength, or certainty, of the expectation of uncontrollability and, in the case of the affective and self-esteem deficits, on the importance of the outcome.

Although this model was derived from experimental studies in the laboratory, it shares several important points of conceptual similarity with theories of depression developed from clinical observation and practice. The psychodynamic conceptualization identifies loss as the central precipitating factor in exogenous depression. In the broadest sense, loss can refer to a real object loss, a symbolic loss, or the loss of hope of fulfilling a fantasy.[39,40] Gaylin[41] summarizes this position as follows (p 390):

What is important to realize is that depression can be precipitated by the loss or removal of anything that the individual over-values in terms of his security. To the extent that one's sense of well-being, safety, or security is dependent on love, money, social position, power, drugs or obsessional defenses—to that extent one will be threatened by its loss. When the reliance is preponderant, the individual despairs of survival and gives up. It is this despair which has been called depression. Hopeless and helpless, he gives up the struggle.

There is always a need for caution in comparing theoretical concepts taken from different frames of reference. However, the concept of loss, as used by the psychodynamic writers, seems to clearly imply elements of uncontrollability in two senses. First, important losses are rarely events that are desired or sought after by an individual. Therefore, the occurrence of a loss is likely to be experienced as uncontrollable since it takes place outside of one's volition. Second, uncontrollability is frequently an aspect of loss in the sense that, once the loss has occurred, the individual may feel powerless to either cope with its consequences or regain what has been lost. Bibring,[42] in particular, has emphasized this experience of powerlessness, or helplessness, as the central feature in depression (pp 162−163):

> In all these instances, the individuals either felt helplessly exposed to superior powers, fatal organic disease, or recurrent neurosis, or to the seemingly inescapable fate of being lonely, isolated, or unloved, or unavoidably confronted with the apparent evidence of being weak, inferior, or a failure. . . . From this point of view, depression can be defined as the emotional expression (indication) of a state of helplessness or powerlessness of the ego, irrespective of what may have caused the breakdown of the mechanism which established his self-esteem.

Beck's cognitive model views depression as fundamentally a disorder of cognition rather than of affect.[43,44] Beck postulates that depression arises when some stressful event, especially one involving loss, activates within the individual a set of depressogenic cognitive schemas involving highly negative views of the self, the world, and the future. While Beck describes a number of types of cognitive distortions seen in depressed patients, many of these distortions relate to pessimistic expectations about the future, a drastically diminished sense of personal competence, and feelings of hopelessness about being able to effect change in one's life. This description is quite similar to the expectancy of uncontrollability which is central to the learned helplessness hypothesis, and both theories share an emphasis on the primary importance of cognitive factors in the etiology and treatment of depression.

While it is encouraging to note these points of conceptual similarity between theories derived from such different backgrounds, we must turn our attention to the existing empirical data in order to evaluate the validity of the learned helplessness model. In the remainder of this chapter, we will be addressing ourselves to the question of whether the laboratory phenomenon of learned helplessness is an appropriate and useful model for naturally occurring depression.

The use of experimental or laboratory models has numerous potential advantages in the study of psychopathology.[45,46] The causal variables responsible for the production of laboratory phenomena are generally better defined and more clearly understood than the factors involved in the occurrence of clinical disorders. Thus, as Buchwald, Coyne, and Cole[45] have pointed out: "An appropriate model can increase the precision of our thinking about the disorder and help us to understand the disorder. In addition, we can use the results of easily conducted laboratory studies to help answer vexing questions about the nature, the etiology, and the alleviation of the disorder" (p 180).

However, the phenomena produced by experimental models are usually analogues of naturally occurring psychopathologies rather than exact replicas.[46] For this reason, an experimental model is only appropriate to the extent that it mimics the particular disorder in question, and its usefulness depends on its ability to generate meaningful directions for research. In the following sections, we will first review the empirical evidence supporting the appropriateness of the learned helplessness model as an analogue of depression. We will then examine one area of research—the relationship of stressful live events to depression—and discuss how learned helplessness theory may help us in understanding this relationship.

Empirical Support for the Learned Helplessness Model

The primary requirement for any experimental model of psychopathology is that it must be able to demonstrate similarities between the model and the natural disorder. Miller, Rosellini, and Seligman provide an extensive discussion of the similarities between learned helplessness and depression,[7] and we will simply summarize the main points of their comparison.

One of the main symptoms of helplessness is passivity. Both humans and animals exposed to uncontrollable stimuli are slower in initiating responses or do not respond at all. This passivity has clear parallels to certain features of depression such as loss of energy, retardation of speech and movement, and inactivity or even immobility. Retardation of responding among depressed patients is supported not only by clinical observation but by empirical studies as well. As compared to normal individuals, depressives generally engage in fewer activities and show reduced interpersonal responding.

The second major effect of uncontrollability is interference with learning that responses are related to outcomes. Such interference may account for some of the deficits in cognitive performance frequently seen in depression, including impairments of memory, concentration, and problem-solving abilities. It may also be an important process in the maintenance of depression. Once depression has developed, this type of cognitive interference may prevent individuals from reestablishing belief in the effectiveness of their own behavior and thus serve to reinforce and perpetuate the expectancy of uncontrollability which initially caused the depression.

The lack of motivation which is so commonly a prominent feature of depression may be directly related to the expectancy of uncontrollability postulated by learned helplessness theory. If one believes outcomes are independent of one's responses, it follows that the motivation to engage in goal-directed behavior will be drastically reduced. We should also mention here that subjective feelings of helplessness, hopelessness, and powerlessness are very commonly reported by depressed patients.

In addition to these behavioral and experiential similarities, research with infrahuman species points to two areas in which physiological similarities between depression and learned helplessness have been found. First, the syndrome of depression often includes physical symptoms such as appetite disturbance and loss of sexual desire. Parallel findings have been obtained in animal studies where it was shown that uncontrollable trauma produced weight loss and disruption of food gathering and sexual behavior. Second, one hypothesis on the biochemistry of the affective disorders suggests that some types of depression are associated with a deficiency of catecholamines, especially norepinephrine, at important receptor sites in the brain.[47] While the available research on learned helplessness is limited, depletion of whole-brain norepinephrine has been found in rats exposed to inescapable shock.[7]

DePue and Monroe, in their evaluation of the learned helplessness model, have emphasized the heterogeneity of clinical manifestations of depression and pointed out the limitations of some of the comparisons discussed above.[48] The interested reader should refer to their excellent article for a more comprehensive discussion of the complex issues involved in doing research on depression. We feel, however, that the demonstrated similarities between depression and learned helplessness are sufficiently well established to allow us to proceed to the second phase of our assessment of the model. Here we wish to examine the following questions: Does the learned helplessness model provide us with hypotheses about depression which are testable in the laboratory and, if so, are these hypotheses supported by the data?

According to the learned helplessness model, naturally occurring depression and laboratory induced helplessness share the central feature of expectations of response-outcome independence. Therefore, the model predicts that depressed subjects and nondepressed subjects who have been made helpless should show the same behavioral deficits relative to normal controls.[49] This prediction has been tested in a number of studies conducted by Seligman and his associates.[50-56] These studies have all employed a 3 (controllability) × 2 (depression) design in which depressed and nondepressed subjects were divided into helpless, nonhelpless, and control groups during the first phase of the standard learned helplessness paradigm. Afterwards, the effects of the helplessness training were assessed by having all of the subjects perform a task where outcomes were controllable.

The results of the studies have consistently shown that nondepressed subjects exposed to uncontrollable outcomes (e.g., inescapable noise or insoluble problems) performed much like depressed subjects not exposed to uncontrollability. In other words, the experimental induction of helplessness with nondepressives produced performance deficits identical to those seen in naturally depressed individuals who had not received helplessness training. Thus, in the second phase of the procedure, the performance of both groups was characterized by failure to learn that their responses were instrumental in controlling what happened to them. The consistency of these findings supports the hypothesis that learned helplessness and naturally occurring depression are parallel phenomena which may share similarities in etiology as well as in symptoms.

A second prediction which can be generated from the learned helplessness model is that depressed subjects and nondepressed helpless subjects should both hold distorted expectancies about their ability to control future outcomes. This prediction has been confirmed by several experimental studies which have demonstrated distorted perceptions on the part of depressed and helpless students.[51,53-56] Nondepressed subjects exposed to inescapable noise perceived reinforcement on a skill task as less response-contingent, relative to subjects exposed to escapable noise or no noise. Depressed subjects not exposed to any helplessness training showed similar distortions. As compared to nondepressed subjects, depressed subjects tended to view their behavior on a skill task as if it were based on chance. Furthermore, Miller, Seligman, and Kurlander found that this perception was specific to depression and did not occur among anxious students.[56] Thus, as was predicted by the learned helplessness model, both depressed and helpless subjects exhibited a tendency to distort their perceptions of skill tasks in the direction of response-outcome independence.

In their reformulation of the learned helplessness model, Abramson et al. suggested that susceptibility to depression should be associated with an attributional style in which the individual tends to attribute failure to global, stable, and internal factors.[29] Several studies have examined subjects' attributions about the causes of their performance and found that depressed students, as compared to nondepressed, were more likely to attribute their failures to internal factors.[52,57,58] However, these studies measured only one of three attributional dimensions believed to be important in depression. Seligman, Abramson, Semmel, and von Baeyer undertook a more comprehensive assessment of attributional style by eliciting students' attributions about twelve hypothetical situations, six describing positive outcomes and six describing negative outcomes.[59] Their findings were consistent with the reformulated model's prediction about attributional style. Relative to nondepressed students, depressed students attributed negative outcomes to global, stable, and internal factors.

In summary, the available empirical evidence concerning behavioral deficits, distorted task perceptions, and attributional style supports the appropriateness and usefulness of the learned helplessness model of depression. At this point, however, we should mention two limitations which must be taken into account in interpreting the existing data. First, as Miller, Rosellini, and Seligman[7] have acknowledged, "the fact that noncontingent reinforcement results in behavioral deficits similar to those of naturally occurring depression does not *prove* that the depression was also produced by experiences with uncontrollable reinforcement" (p 123). Studies such as those described in the preceding sections provide growing support for the hypothesis that learned helplessness and depression are parallel phenomena, but it is likely that the etiological factors proposed by the model are relevant only to certain groups of naturally occurring depression.

The second limitation we wish to point out is a methodological one concerning the criteria used for identifying depressed populations. To date, the vast majority of learned helplessness research has used college students as subjects and divided them into depressed and nondepressed groups according to their scores on standard self-rating instruments, generally the Beck Depression Inventory.[43] DePue and Monroe have discussed in considerable detail the problems associated with this approach,[48] and we would like to emphasize two of the issues they raised. First, scales such as the BDI were designed for use in assessing the severity of depressive symptoms and are not valid instruments for differential diagnosis. As a result, the depressed groups used in learned helplessness research are likely to be extremely heterogeneous and it is not known how comparable these subjects are to individuals with clinical diagnoses of depression. The second issue is a closely related one and involves the nature of mild depressive states. It is unclear whether mild and severe forms of depression are best thought of as qualitatively distinct phenomena or as extreme points on a continuum. Thus, findings obtained with a nonclinical, mildly depressed population may not be generalizable to clinically depressed patients. For these reasons, DePue and Monroe and

Buchwald, Coyne, and Cole[45] have recommended that future research on learned helplessness exercise greater precision in the selection and description of depressed subjects.

Learned Helplessness, Depression and Stressful Life Events

So far, research on learned helplessness and depression has taken the approach of exposing depressed and nondepressed subjects to the learned helplessness procedure, and comparing the responses of the two groups. As noted above, such an approach has its limitations as well as its advantages. An alternative strategy for research would be to select a well defined group of clinically depressed individuals and to examine how the learned helplessness model can add to our understanding of the phenomena associated with naturally occurring depression. The results of this type of research could provide a valuable complement to the findings of laboratory studies and increase our confidence in the usefulness of the model.

Since the learned helplessness model is most clearly relevant to reactive depressions, the study of life events and depression seems to be one area of research in which the model could be applied quite productively. The relationship of stressful life events to the onset of depression has been the subject of considerable controversy.[60,61] Even where the data show a definite association between these two factors, the nature of the causal role of life events remains uncertain.

We believe that hypotheses derived from the learned helplessness model may be valuable in clarifying the relationship between depression and life events. The model predicts that it is not stressful events per se, but uncontrollable events which are most likely to produce depression.[7] This prediction suggests an additional dimension—namely, perceived controllability—which may be crucial in understanding the impact of stressful life events.

Paykel has conducted extensive field studies with clinically depressed patients which are relvant for consideration here.[61-63] Using a retrospective approach to life events, he compared the depressives with a group of individuals suffering from other psychiatric disorders in terms of the number of life events they reported as having preceded the onset of a psychiatric episode.

Paykel found that the depressed patients reported significantly larger numbers of life events than did the nondepressives. Depressives were also found to report more "exits from the social field", a category of events dealing with terminations of social interactions (e.g., death of a family member, divorce, having a child leave home). As we mentioned in our discussion of psychodynamic theories, important losses seem to implicitly contain elements of uncontrollability. Thus, Paykel's findings may be interpreted as consistent with the learned helplessness prediction concerning uncontrollable events.

The results of Kobasa's recent study on stressful life events among middle and upper level executives are also supportive of learned helplessness theory.[64] She found that executives who experienced high stress but little illness showed a significantly greater sense of personal control over their lives when compared to executives who reported high levels of illness in response to high stress. However, Kobasa conceptualized control as a personality dimension rather than as an aspect of the subjects' perceptions of events.

A series of pilot studies conducted by Hiroto focused directly on the perceived controllability of life events as a contributing factor to the onset of acute depression.[65] A total of twelve adult psychiatric outpatients from the University of California Medical Center in San Francisco underwent an extensive interview about life events which had occurred from one to six months prior to their first subjective feelings of distress. The sample included six reactive depressives and six nondepressed patients, the latter group representing a variety of diagnoses such as adjustment reactions, marital maladjustments, and so forth.

In the interview, the controllability of each reported life event was assessed along the following four dimensions: the predictability of the event's occurrence; the predictability of the termination and/or consequences of the event; the desirability of the outcome; and efforts made to alter the event. As predicted, the depressed patients, relative to the nondepressives, reported significantly more uncontrollable life events in the period just prior to the onset of disturbance.

We have just begun a study which will attempt to replicate these findings with a large sample of male psychiatric inpatients. As in Hiroto's pilot studies, patients are interviewed about important life events which occurred just prior to their first subjective feelings of distress, and the perceived controllability of these events is assessed along a number of dimensions. In keeping with the reformulated model of learned helplessness, we are also eliciting patients' causal attributions for each event. We predict that depressed patients will report more uncontrollable life events than patients who are not depressed and that the depressives' attributions about events will be more internal, stable, and global.

A unique feature of this study is that it includes a laboratory procedure in addition to the above mentioned interview, and the same subjects are being used in both phases of the study. Several days before being interviewed, each patient participates in a standard learned helplessness procedure involving exposure to either soluble or insoluble cognitive problems. As part of this procedure, patients are asked for their attributions regarding the causes of their success or failure in solving the problems. Thus we will be able to assess the degree of similarity between an individual's attributions about important life events and his attributions about his performance in the laboratory.

CONCLUSIONS AND RECOMMENDATIONS

Learned helplessness is one example of a laboratory model which has been used extensively in the study of psychopathology, and it has generated a sizeable body of research in a relatively short period of time. So far research efforts have been directed primarily towards validating the appropriateness of learned helplessness as a model of depression. Clearly this is the first and most essential task in the development of such a model, and the process involved is similar to that of construct validation.[66] Since a construct, by definition, cannot be measured directly, its validity is established by progressively building up a network of empirical findings which support the construct and rule out alternative explanations.

In our evaluation of the learned helplessness model of depression, we have tried to establish such a network. We first described the conceptual parallels between the learned helplessness model and other theories of depression and reviewed the similarities between helplessness deficits and various depressive symptoms. We then presented empirical evidence which confirms several of the model's predictions about depression and discussed how learned helplessness theory could be applied to the study of stressful life events. On the whole, the existing research supports the appropriateness of learned helplessness as a model of depression and suggests that this is a promising area for continued investigation.

However as we noted previously, research on learned helplessness and depression has generally been conducted within the narrow confines of the laboratory experiment, using college students as subjects. We feel there is a great need to broaden the focus of research both by extending our studies to a variety of populations and by applying the model to areas outside of the laboratory. In particular, the following questions need to be addressed in future research:

1.   What type of depression does learned helplessness model?

Since most of the published studies have used the Beck Depression Inventory as the sole measure of depression, we cannot say at this point whether their findings are relevant to depression as a distinct and clearly defined clinical disorder or only to depression as a general affective-cognitive state which may coexist with a variety of other physical and psychiatric disorders. Along similar lines, DePue and Monroe have pointed out that the category of "reactive depressions" includes situational, minor, and major depressive disorders.[48] They suggest the need for distinguishing and redefining the etiological role of learned helplessness in each of these types of depression. It is important, therefore, that more research be done with individuals who have received a definite and reliable diagnosis of clinical depression, and that all studies attempt a more precise specification of the type of depressed subjects being used.

2. Are the deficits predicted by the learned helplessness model specific to depression, or are they a general feature of psychopathology?

Again, research on clinical populations is necessary in order to answer this question. Some initial support for the specificity of the model was found in a recent study by Abramson et al.[50] which used four subject groups: depressed nonschizophrenics (unipolar depressives), depressed schizophrenics, nondepressed schizophrenics, and normal controls. The results indicated that only the unipolar depressives exhibited distorted perceptions of response-outcome independence on skill and chance tasks. The depressed and nondepressed schizophrenics did not differ from the normal controls in their task perceptions. This study exemplifies the type of research needed in this area, and it is recommended that additional studies be done to evaluate the specificity of the learned helplessness model to depression.

3. Are there individual differences which affect susceptibility to learned helplessness?

Research with animals has shown that dogs raised singly in cages are more susceptible to the effects of uncontrollable shock than dogs of unknown history.[12] Miller, Rosellini, and Seligman suggested that the cage-reared dogs were more vulnerable because they had been deprived of opportunities to learn that they could master their environments.[7] But research on human helplessness has directed little attention to individuals differences in susceptibility. Extrapolating from the animal research, one might predict that individuals who have experienced mastery and competence in their lives would be less vulnerable to the effects of helplessness training than persons who have little sense of mastery over their environment. In our current research project, we are assessing patients' previous experiences of competence in various areas of their lives (e.g., academic achievement, interpersonal relationships, work performance), and we plan to examine whether differences along this dimension are associated with differential susceptibility to helplessness effects. The concept of attributional style recently proposed by Seligman et al.[59] is another factor which may be related to individual differences in vulnerability.

4. What is the relationship between causal attributions and subsequent behavior?

The reformulated model of Abramson et al.[29] proposes that an individual exposed to an uncontrollable event makes an attribution about the cause of the event and that this attribution then determines his or her response. Wortman and Dintzer contend that the link between attribution and behavior is not as straightforward as the model implies.[67] They suggest instead that the individual may develop several hypotheses about the cause of the event and that subsequent behavior may be directed largely towards information gathering and hypothesis testing. Similarly, the relationship between attributions and affect is presently unclear, especially concerning the direction of causality involved. As Wortman and Dintzer[67] ask: "Are certain attributional styles more likely to result in depression than others? Or does depressed affect determine the way attributions are made?" (p 86). There is a definite need for further research on these issues, and Hammen and her associates are presently conducting several longitudinal studies designed to clarify the relationship of stressful events and attributions to subsequent affective responses and coping behavior.[68]

5. What implications does learned helplessness research have for the treatment of depressed patients?

This is a crucial issue since it bridges the gap between clinical research and practice. Klein and Seligman have demonstrated the "reversal" of laboratory-induced helplessness deficits in college students,[51] but the applicability of these findings to the individual treatment of depressed patients is yet to be determined. As the parallels between learned helplessness and depression become more firmly established, such studies may be helpful in suggesting new treatment procedures or in evaluating the effective components of existing therapies. In our opinion, learned helplessness theory also has more immediate implications for developing treatment strategies on broader levels, such as the therapeutic milieu. For example, recent studies by Langer and Rodin[33] and by Schultz[34] have highlighted the importance of personal control and responsibility for the psychological well-being of the institutionalized aged.

In conclusion, we believe that these questions raise critical issues for the future development of learned helplessness theory. At present the theory has demonstrated considerable heuristic value in stimulating experimental research on the effects of uncontrollable events and the relationship of such events to naturally occurring depressions. Much of this research has been directed towards evaluating the adequacy of the learned helplessness model as an analogue of depression. The availability of a valid and appropriate laboratory model affords us greater precision in investigating the interplay of life experiences and psychological processes involved in the onset and maintenance of depressive states. It is hoped that continued systematic study of laboratory induced helplessness and naturally occurring depression will contribute to the development of more effective treatments for this most common of psychiatric disorders.

REFERENCES

1. Bowlby J: Separation (vol 2 of Attachment and Loss). New York, Basic Books, 1973
2. Spitz RA: Anaclitic depression, in Freud A, Hartmann H, Kris E (eds): Psychoanal Study Child (vol 2). New York, International University Press, 1946
3. Spitz RA: Hospitalism: An inquiry into the genesis of psychiatric conditions in early childhood, in Freud A, Hartmann H, Kris, E (eds): Psychoanal Study Child (vol 1). New York, International University Press, 1945
4. Williams TA, Friedman RJ, Secunda SK: The depressive illness (special report). Washington, D.C.: Ntl Inst Mental Health, 1970
5. Seligman MEP: Helplessness: On depression, development, and death. San Francisco, W.H. Freeman and Company, 1975
6. Seligman MEP, Klein DC, Miller WR: Depression, in Leitenberg H (ed): Handbook of behavior modification and behavior therapy. Englewood Cliffs, Prentice Hall, 1976
7. Miller WR, Rosellini RA, Seligman MEP: Learned helplessness and depression, in Maser JD, Seligman MEP (eds): Psychopathology: Experimental models. San Francisco, Freeman, 1977
8. Overmier JB, Seligman MEP: Effects of inescapable shock upon subsequent escape and avoidance learning. J Comp Phys Psychol 62:28−33, 1967
9. Seligman MEP, Maier SF: Failure to escape traumatic shock. J Exp Psychol 74:1−9, 1967
10. Maier SF, Seligman MEP, Solomon RL: Pavlovian fear conditioning and learned helplessness, in Campbell B, Church R (eds): Punishment. New York, Appleton-Century-Crofts, 1969
11. Maier SF, Seligman MEP: Learned helplessness: Theory and evidence. J Exp Psychol 105:3−46, 1976
12. Seligman MEP, Groves D: Nontransient learned helplessness. Psychon Sci 19:191−192, 1970
13. Seligman MEP: Learned helplessness. Ann Rev Med 23:407−412, 1972
14. Braud W, Wepman B, Russo P: Task and species generality of the ''helplessness'' phenomenon. Psychon Sci 16:154−155, 1969
15. Hiroto DS: Locus of control and learned helplessness. J Exp Psychol 102:187−193, 1974
16. Rotter JB: Generalized expectancies for internal versus external control of reinforcement. Psychol Monogr 80 (1, #609), 1966

17. Hiroto DS, Seligman MEP: Generality of learned helplessness in man. J Person Soc Psychol 31:311–327, 1975

18. Cohen S, Rothbart M, Phillips S: Locus of control and the generality of learned helplessness in humans. J Person Soc Psychol 34:1049–1056, 1976

19. Dweck CS: The role of expectations and attributions in the alleviation of learned helplessness. J Person Soc Psychol 31:674–685, 1975

20. Dweck CS, Reppucci N: Learned helplessness and reinforcement responsibility in children. J Person Soc Psychol 25:109–116, 1973

21. Griffiths M: Effects of non-contingent success and failure on mood and performance. J Person 45:442–457, 1977

22. Roth S: The effects of experimentally induced expectancies of control: Facilitation of controlling behavior or learned helplessness. Unpublished doctoral dissertation, Northwestern Univ., 1973

23. Roth S: A revised model of learned helplessness in humans. J Pers 48:103–133, 1980

24. Roth S, Bootzin RR: Effects of experimentally induced expectancies of external control: An investigation of learned helplessness. J Person Soc Psychol 29:253–264, 1974

25. Roth S, Kilpatrick-Tabak B: Developments in the study of learned helplessness in humans: A critical review. Unpublished manuscript, Duke Univ., 1977

26. Roth S, Kubal L: Effects of noncontingent reinforcement on tasks of differing importance: Facilitation and learned helplessness. J Person Soc Psychol 32:680–691, 1975

27. Thornton JW, Jacobs PD: Learned helplessness in human subjects. J Exp Psychol 87:369–372, 1971

28. Miller IW, Gold J: The relationship of percentage of reinforcement and situational importance in the development of learned helplessness. Unpublished manuscript, Brown University, 1978

29. Abramson LY, Seligman, MEP, Teasdale J: Learned helplessness in humans: Critique and reformulation. J Abn Psychol 87:49–74, 1978

30. Weiner B: Theories of motivation: From mechanism to cognition. Chicago, Rand McNally, 1972

31. Weiner B (ed): Achievement motivation and attribution theory. Morristown, NJ, General Learning Press, 1974

32. Weiner B, Russell D, Lerman D: Affective consequences of causal ascriptions, in Harvey JH, Ickes WJ, Kidd RF (eds): New directions in attribution research (vol 2). Hillsdale, NJ, Lawrence Erlbaum, 1978

33. Langer EJ, Rodin J: The effects of choice and enhanced personal responsibility for the aged: A field experiment in an institutional setting. J Person Soc Psychol 34:191–199, 1976

34. Schultz R: Effects of control and predictability on the physical and psychological well-being of the institutionalized aged. J Person Soc Psychol 33:563–574, 1976

35. Krantz DS, Glass DC, Snyder ML: Helplessness, stress levels, and the coronary prone behavior pattern. J Exp Soc Psychol 10:284–300, 1974

36. Krantz DS, Glass DC: Environmental control and pattern A behavior. Unpublished manuscript, Univ. of Texas at Austin, 1974

37. Glass DC, Singer J: Urban stress: Experiments on noise and social stressors. New York, Academic Press, 1972
38. Rodin J: Density, perceived choice, and response to controllable and uncontrollable outcomes. J Exp Soc Psychol 12:564−579, 1976
39. White RB, Gilliland RM: Elements of psychopathology: The mechanisms of defense. New York, Grune & Stratton, 1975
40. White RB, Davis HK, Cantrell WA: Psychodynamics of depression: Implications for treatment, in Usdin G (ed): Depression: Clinical, biological, and psychological perspectives. New York, Brunner/Mazel, 1978
41. Gaylin W (ed): The meaning of despair. New York, Science, 1968.
42. Bibring E: The mechanism of depression, in Gaylin W (ed): The meaning of despair. New York, Science, 1968
43. Beck AT: Depression: Clinical, experimental, and theoretical aspects. New York, Hoeber, 1967
44. Beck AT: Cognitive therapy and emotional disorders. New York, International University, 1976
45. Buchwald AM, Coyne JC, Cole CS: A critical evaluation of the learned helplessness model of depression. J Abn Psychol 87:180−193, 1978
46. Abramson LY, Seligman MEP: Modeling psychopathology in the laboratory: History and rationale, in Maser JD, Seligman MEP (eds): Psychopathology: Experimental models. San Francisco, Freeman, 1977
47. Schildkraut J: Neuropsychopharmacology and the affective disorders. Boston, Little Brown, 1970
48. DePue RA, Monroe SM: Learned helplessness in the perspective of the depressive disorders: Conceptual and definitional issues. J Abn Psychol 87:3−20, 1978
49. Seligman MEP: Comment and integration. J Abn Psychol 87:165−179, 1978
50. Abramson LY, Garber J, Edwards NB, Seligman MEP: Expectancy changes in depression and schizophrenia. J Abn Psychol 87:102−109, 1978
51. Klein DC, Seligman MEP: Reversal of performance deficits in learned helplessness and depression. J Abn Psychol 85:11−26, 1976
52. Klein DC, Fencil-Morse E, Seligman MEP: Learned helplessness, depression, and the attribution of failure. J Person Soc Psychol 33:508−516, 1976
53. Miller WR, Seligman MEP: Depression and the perception of reinforcement. J Abn Psychol 82:62−73, 1973
54. Miller WR, Seligman MEP: Depression and learned helplessness in man. J Abn Psychol 84:228−238, 1975
55. Miller WR, Seligman MEP: Learned helplessness, depression, and the perception of reinforcement. Behav Res Ther 14:7−17, 1976
56. Miller WR, Seligman MEP, Kurlander HM: Learned helplessness, depression, and anxiety. J Nerv Men Dis 161:347−357, 1975
57. Rizley R: Depression and distortion in the attribution of causality. J Abn Psychol 87:32−48, 1978
58. Kupier NA: Depression and causal attributions for success and failure. J Person Soc Psychol 36:236−246, 1978
59. Seligman MEP, Abramson LY, Semmel A, von Baeyer C: Depressive attributional style. J Abn Psychol 88:242−247, 1979

60. Brown GW: Life-events and the onset of depressive and schizophrenic conditions, in Gunderson EKE, Rahe RH (eds): Life stress and illness. Springfield, Ill, Thomas, 1974

61. Paykel ES: Recent life events and clinical depression, in Gunderson EKE, Rahe RH (eds): Life stress and illness. Springfield, Ill, Thomas, 1974

62. Paykel ES, Myers JK, Klerman GL, et al: Life events and depression: A controlled study. Arch Gen Psych 21:753−760, 1969

63. Paykel ES: Life events and acute depressions, in Scott JP, Seray EC (eds): Separation and depression. Washington, DC: Amer Assoc Advanc of Science, 1973

64. Kobasa SC: Stressful life events, personality and health: An inquiry into hardiness. J Person Soc Psychol 37:1−11, 1979

65. Hiroto DS: Learned helplessness: From the laboratory to the field. Southw. Rocky Mtn. meeting of the Amer Assoc Adv Science, Los Alamos, New Mexico, 1975

66. Cronbach LJ, Meehl, PE: Construct validity in psychological tests. Psychol Bull 52:281−302, 1955

67. Wortman CB, Dintzer L: Is an attributional analysis of the learned helplessness phenomenon viable?: A critique of the Abramson-Seligman-Teasdale reformulation. J Abn Psychol 87:75−90, 1978

68. Hammen CL: personal communication. May, 1979

Kenneth S. Pope

10
Clinical Psychology: Coordinating Therapy and Research

Relating research to clinical practice is a difficult topic for most biobehavioral scientists to address. Though many clinical psychologists embrace the Boulder model of being a "scientist-practitioner", a realistic look at the profession suggests that most psychologists, through frustration, are abandoning this ideal in practice, if not in theory. People trained in clinical psychology are defining themselves more and more as either researchers or psychotherapists. The high divorce rate between research and practice is not without some mutual recriminations. Researchers charge that most psychotherapy (as well as psychological testing and other clinical work) does not rest upon a sound scientific basis, but seems more like an art, a religion, or just downright huckstering. Clinicians counter by characterizing most research as trivial, artificial, and useless to the practitioner.

This chapter will focus on three research projects, each concerned with a different aspect of clinical practice. The first concerns setting the conditions for practice; the specific topic is the relationship of fees to psychotherapy. The second concerns determining the content or ideals of practice; the specific topic is the day-to-day flow of human consciousness. The third concerns preparing those who practice; the topic is sexual intimacy in psychology training programs. Each project suggests a common difficulty in conducting research which both grows out of the practitioner's concerns and produces findings which can successfully guide future clinical practice.

SETTING THE CONDITIONS FOR PRACTICE: FEES
AND PSYCHOTHERAPY

As a graduate student, and intern learning to do psychotherapy, I was struck by the frequent assertions in the literature that the fees for psychotherapy should be high. Part of what made this interesting was that while such statements were common among the theory, or "how to do it" literature, the subject of paying for therapy was almost totally absent from the research literature. My colleagues—Leland Wilkinson and Jesse Geller—and I were able to locate only four studies of the effects of fees upon therapy, and each of these contained serious methodological flaws (e.g., no control of such potentially confounding variables as socioeconomic status and diagnosis, small sample size, nonquantifiable results).[1,4] The studies yielded contradictory findings.

Another part of what made interesting these assertions that therapy should cost a lot was the rationale: charging large fees is good for the patients; but this, they claim, is not done from greed, self-interest, or the fact that they have trained hard and long in order to be able to offer a valuable skill. Rather, this is done for the good of the patient: the patient will not complete successfully, nor benefit from therapy unless he or she is paying a lot of money. This rationale can be traced to Freud, who believed that "The value of the treatment is not enhanced in the patient's eyes if a very low fee is asked . . . The absence of the regulating effect offered by the payment of a fee makes itself very painfully felt; the whole relationship is removed from the real world, and the patient is deprived of a strong motive for endeavoring to bring the treatment to an end."[5] Menninger felt that "The analysis will not go well if the patient is paying less than he can reasonably afford to pay. It should be a definite sacrifice for him."[6] Kubie stood behind a strict fee system, including full payment for both missed and cancelled appointments. "If the patient were not charged for appointments which he missed, the analyst would in effect be offering him a financial inducement to escape painful sessions, since he could go off and enjoy himself and save money as well."[7] Assertions that the fee itself was therapeutic or a necessary condition of therapy were common in the writings not only of psychoanalysts and psychodynamically-oriented therapists, but also those of other orientations. Cognitive dissonance, for instance, was employed by Davids to support the notion that "In order to accomplish any significant therapeutic work the patient must be charged a fee that is somewhat painful and discomforting."[8]

But do most psychotherapists who are currently practicing endorse such assertions that the fee has therapeutic effects? To find out, my colleagues and I conducted a national survey (after a pilot survey in New Haven) in which a questionnaire was sent to a random sample of 500 psychiatrists, 250 clinical psychologists, and 250 social workers listed in the national professional directories. The final sample included 446 anonymous replies, or a 45 percent return. Respondents provided professional information about themselves and indicated the degree to which they agreed or disagreed with each of 29 assertions concerning fee assessment for psychotherapy. Although each of the 29 assertions elicited the full range of agreements and disagreements, this survey provides evidence of a widespread belief in the therapeutic effects of fees.[9]

To what extent does this belief, which finds expression in the fee assessment policies of many mental health organizations and private practitioners, find support from research? As noted earlier, there were few empirical studies. To gather more substantial evidence, Pope, Geller, and Wilkinson gathered data from the records of 434 clients who had received individual outpatient therapy at the Connecticut Mental Health Center in 1972.[10] The three predictor variables were fee (no payment, welfare, insurance, scaled payment, and full payment), diagnosis (psychosis, neurosis, personality disorder, transient situational disturbance, and other), and socioeconomic status (five levels). A least-squares multivariate analysis of variance found only diagnosis to be significantly related to the outcome, number of appointments, and attendance of individual outpatient psychotherapy. Though numerous subtests were conducted (for instance, using as a sample only those who were diagnosed as neurotic, or only those in the lowest SES group), there was simply no evidence of significant effects of fee assessment categories on the therapeutic process. Balch, Ireland, and Lewis in a replication of this study in a different setting found no relation between fees and measure of psychotherapy outcome.[11]

The issue of fees and psychotherapy raises some questions regarding the relationship between research and practice and suggests a potential source of difficulty in constructing a bridge between the two. Given the prevalence of the fee issue in the theoretical writings of practitioners and the widespread belief among practitioners in the therapeutic efficacy of fees, why has so little research been generated? And the other side of the coin: given the paucity of research evidence supporting the efficacy of fees and the fact that the more rigorously designed studies fail to show any effect of fee upon the process or outcome of therapy, why does fee-setting practice continue to be based upon this belief? A major source of difficulty may be that the amount of money paid for therapy (regardless of whether it comes directly from the client or from third-party sources) affects the livelihood of many mental health organizations and individual practitioners. It is difficult to maintain a disinterested stance regarding an issue which directly affects the ability of those of us who are at one end of the continuum to put groceries on the table, or those of us at the other end to put a second car in the garage which is situated next to the swimming pool which we use when we're not on vacation in Aruba. As with the fee issue in particular, so it is with more general issues: we may experience a reluctance to undertake certain research, or to incorporate the findings of research into practice, when the certain, likely, or in some cases even possible result will be less income (or security, or status, or power, etc.). We may be less than eager to hear that people with emotional or behavioral problems may receive help more effectively, more efficiently, more equitably, or more economically than the help which we are personally able to provide. It is at these uncomfortable times that we begin talking of the overwhelming complexity of human life (which is to say, our own clinical experience), of the inestimable value of clinical experience (which is to say, our own clinical experience), or simply change the subject. Rarely, in such circumstances, are we prompted to reaffirm the value of research and the beneficial effects of a close interplay between research and practice.

DETERMINING THE CONTENT OF PRACTICE: THE NORMAL FLOW OF CONSCIOUSNESS

The practitioner inevitably makes assumptions—however implicit, however discrepant from what the client is saying or otherwise conveying—about what that client is experiencing from moment to moment, and about the importance, or perhaps lack of importance, of that experience to the therapeutic enterprise. Yet normal, day-to-day consciousness was long neglected by psychological research.

Soon after the turn of the century, psychology took a behavioristic turn, so sharply that serious investigation of the flow of human consciousness was left behind. "In 1913 John Watson mercifully closed the bloodshot inner eye of American psychology. With great relief the profession trained its exteroceptors on the laboratory animal."[12] Even Freudian thought and related movements, with their emphasis on the interior life of the individual, created little empirical knowledge of the movement of conscious experience because they emphasized the overwhelming power of the unconscious and represented the person's life as determined by a hydraulic-like system of drives of which the individual was often unaware.

This tendency to act as if human consciousness were virtually nonexistent had some amazing consequences. The clinical practitioner, seeking empirically-based theory to supplement his or her own clinical observations, would consult textbooks on thinking[13,14] and find little or nothing about the flow of consciousness and imagination, would examine books on personality[15] and adolescence[16] and discover little on daydreaming or fantasy. In spite of a recent reawakening interest in the stream of consciousness, major figures in psychological research still lament the "diverting preoccupation with a supposed or real inner life."[17]

The experimental investigations of consciousness which have been undertaken in the last decade or so have generally focused upon the outcome of specific directed thinking tasks or upon isolated, static aspects of thought (for example, the time it takes to rotate mentally a geometric form; the effectiveness of imagery in paired-associate learning; comparing the size of real or imagined wooden balls; the vividness of imagined visual scenes as a factor in systematic desensitization). The emergent picture of thought process, therefore, often possesses a quality of organization and rationality that is hard to reconcile with the nature of the flow of consciousness as it is presented by artists or with our own stream of consciousness if we observe it in its natural course.

An additional factor enters in: as scientific researchers, we value rational, "secondary-process" thought processes, and the fact that we are greatly dependent on published writings for the communication and dissemination of our ideas tends to increase our contact with (and perhaps our valuing of) thought that is sequential, logical, analytic, and verbal.

The professional writings, then, tend to view consciousness as primarily tied in to here-and-now, task-oriented, secondary-process activities. What Freud referred to as "primary-process" thought (distant memories, fleeting images, imaginary anticipations of the future, fantasies) is seen as either taking up what little space is left over after our real thinking is done, or else as intrusively interfering with that real thinking. Such primary-process thought (which in this context connotes more primitive thinking) is generally considered to be regressive, even though later apologists, such as Kris, tried to put a good light on the whole affair by saying that good consequences were possible when there was "regression in the service of the ego."[18] Nevertheless, the frequent indulgence in fantasy, daydreaming, or nonsecondary-process thinking is often construed as pathological, though there has been little research basis for this view.

Building on the work of others in this area,[19-21] I undertook an investigation of the flow of consciousness of 90 presumably normal people, half of them women, half men. The idea was to see what types of thoughts passed through people's minds when they were not given artificial or experimental directed thinking tasks; I wanted a picture of thought that is closer to our normal, day-to-day flow of awareness. Each person reported his or her stream of consciousness in a variety of conditions (alone or with someone else present; sitting, lying down, walking around). Many of the participants recorded their experiences by speaking into a portable tape recorder. The transcripts of these recordings were then analyzed along a number of dimensions, each analysis being considered potentially worthwhile only if a pair of independent judges reached a sufficiently high level of agreement, both with each other and with the participant (who was asked to analyze his or her transcript). And yet, participants in the pilot study reported some difficulty using the technique: often the flow of consciousness proceeded too fast for them to keep up with in a verbal narrative, or else their moment-to-moment experience was simply too difficult to translate into words. So a second technique of reporting was devised. Participants carried a small key-press in their hands, and a record of their operation of these devices was made on a cumulative recorder. Participants were asked to press the key to indicate relatively simple aspects of the stream of thought (for example, whenever a shift in the content of their consciousness occurred, or whenever their stream of thought was predominantly concerned with something in the current, immediate environment).

The results of this study suggest that many aspects of the flow of consciousness (such as the proportion of time spent with consciousness primarily focused on the current, immediate environment; or the frequency with which our thoughts shift from one subject to another) vary systematically in relation to specifiable conditions (such as solitude or posture).[22] More relevant to the preceeding discussion, this study and similar ones[23,24] suggest that the normal, day-to-day flow of consciousness is more characterized by primary-process than by secondary-process thought, and that our thoughts are more oriented toward long-term memory or future fantasy than to here-and-now, task-oriented material. Furthermore, the research provided no evidence that those who engaged most in fantasy and daydreaming showed any more anxiety, depression, or other characteristics often considered pathological or at least undesirable.

The practitioner's longstanding difficulty in finding much research data on the flow of consciousness that relates directly to the day-to-day experience of either clinician or client, that can be translated directly into clinical work, suggests another fairly obvious source of difficulty in the dialogue between research and practice. As researchers, we find ourselves not only bound to study only what it is possible to study (given our technology, methodology, funding, and time) but also drawn to study what is personally convenient to study. On a large scale, behaviorism, for all of its beneficial contributions, had the side-effect that we not only set aside, for a long while, the study of anything that could not be directly observed, but also that we denied the importance and sometimes even the existence of what could not be directly observed. Which lead to some fairly bizarre behavior, even for psychologists. Some behaviorists, for instance, claiming to recognize as important only that which could be observed, undertook to treat phobias through systematic desensitization by instructing the client: "Now, I want you to relax and imagine in your mind's eye the image of a snake . . ."

On a more personal scale, we may find it difficult to go beyond our own laboratories, our easily available research participants, our familiar set of experimental manipulations or tests and inventories which, as the advertisements constantly remind us, are easy to administer, score, and interpret.

Perhaps the increasing sophistication and availability of computer technology has also had its disappointing side-effects. No longer confined to studying a few variables which careful reasoning, prior research, or first-hand experience suggest are important, we now can make up, in quantity of variables, what we lose in quality. It is now relatively easy to collect a great many presumably independent and dependent variables from an overwhelming variety of checklists, tests, protocols, inventories (with pressure to select the ever-present short form), and just plain numbers to feed into hungry computers. Trying to end this section on a happier note, we can at least speculate that these developments may have drastically reduced, for all but the most incurably lazy among us, the need to fake data.

PREPARING THOSE WHO PRACTICE: SEXUAL INTIMACY IN TRAINING PROGRAMS

The research project which I have been involved with for a longer time than any other I got the idea for when I was an undergraduate. In that setting, and in each university or training setting I've been associated with since, there's been gossip about what students were sleeping with what teachers. The subject was never discussed in an open, formal forum, but the informal talk of students had its share of rumor, accusation, confession, dramatic narrative, and innuendo. At times, certain teachers were characterized as lecherous, exploitative, and threatening: if the student did not come across with sexual favors, dire consequences would follow in terms of exam grades, dissertation evaluations, letters of recommendation, and job possibilities. Such threats were characterized as being hinted at rather than presented in written, contractual form. At times, certain students were characterized as seductive, exploitative, and manipulative: sexual favors or simple affection was offered in exchange for academic gain. At times, certain sexual relationships between students and teachers were characterized as the sudden blossoming of love, and at other times, intercourse and other sexual intimacies were characterized as simply the casual interaction of two consenting adults, totally irrelevant to the educational enterprise. And at still other times, sexual relations were characterized as part of the education, part of the student's coming to know him or herself, learning to be at ease with intimacy and one's body, learning to explore other people, learning how to reach out and how to be vulnerable. All of which adds up to a lot of times.

In any event, there seemed to be no research whatsoever in this area. Psychologists who had researched with enthusiasm everything, from the topology of pigeon pecks to elevator behavior to preference for button size, had not even approached this topic. Whether such sexual relationships actually occurred, or existed only in gossip, whether they exerted positive, negative, or no effects whatsoever on the training of personal life of psychologists—these were questions for which there were no research data. Indeed, they seemed not even to be recognized as questions: there was no mention of them in the literature on education and training. Standards and guidelines which made clear statements regarding both the rights of students and the issues of sexual behavior (for example, prohibiting sexual relations between therapist and client), were silent on this issue.

In the summer of 1978, Hanna Levenson, Leslie Schover, and I mailed out a questionnaire to 1,000 people (500 males, 500 females) whose names and addresses were listed in the 1977 American Psychological Association Directory Psychotherapy Division 29. This division was selected because it includes not only therapists (for comparison to previous therapist surveys) but also psychologists presumably interested in and aware of psychotherapy training, and with some likelihood of having served as a clinical supervisor, teacher, or administrator. The results are based on replies from 220 women, 245 men, and 16 who did not indicate gender.

In summary of findings my colleagues and I have reported elsewhere,[25] slightly less than 10 percent of the respondents reported sexual contact as students with their educators. Only 3 percent of the males reported such contact, compared with almost 17 percent of the females. The more recent the Ph.D. degree, the more likely a report of experiencing sexual contact with an educator while earning that degree. One-fourth of all recent female graduates (six years or less) reported sexual contact with an educator. Twenty percent of the respondents who indicated some profession (educators or therapists) reported having sexual contact with their students or clients. Whereas women reported more sexual contact as graduate students, it was the men (30 percent) rather than the women (9 percent) who reported significantly more sexual contact as psychologists with their students and clients.

Only 2 percent of those surveyed responded affirmatively to the statement: "I believe that sexual relationships between students and their psychology teachers, administrators, or clinical supervisors can be beneficial to both parties." Seven percent of those indicating that they had practiced psychotherapy reported engaging in sexual contact with their clients. Fourteen percent of the men and 60 percent of the women reported having had a seductive psychology professor, administrator, or clinical supervisor during their years as graduate students.

The lack of research in this area, or even of theoretical discussion, upon which sound policies and procedures for training future practitioners could be based, suggests a third fairly obvious source of difficulty in undertaking research that can guide and inform practice. This is our own discomfort with particular topics. Part of the discomfort may lie in the anticipated political consequences (to our career advancement, perhaps, or to our reputation and sources of referrals for patients) of undertaking or being associated with research on such topics. But another large part may lie with our more direct discomfort with the topic itself. Sexuality has historically been a somewhat troublesome issue. Only with the pioneering efforts of Kinsey, and Masters and Johnson was the topic granted scientific respectability, then to gain rapid popular respectability through the David Reubin phenomenon. Most sex therapists have now identified anxiety about or preoccupation with specific standards of performance as the source of most sexual dysfunction. Human sexuality, they proclaim, has absolutely nothing to do with such standards, and the quicker we can discard such crippling standards altogether, the quicker we can get on with the noncriterion-oriented enjoyment, communication, exploration, sharing, and intimacy that is sexuality. The practitioners of sex therapy are amazingly effective in their work with clients. Ironically, their research demonstrated that clients, after therapy, are much more able to achieve such specific standards of performance.

REFERENCES

1. Koren K, Joyce J: The treatment implications of payment of fees in a clinic setting. Am J of Orthopsych 23:350−357, 1953
2. Schjelderup H: Lasting effects of psychoanalytic treatment. Psychiatry 18:109−133, 1955
3. Lorand S, Console, W: Therapeutic results in psychoanalytic treatment without fee (observation on therapeutic results). Int J Psychoan 39:59−65, 1958
4. Goodman N: Are there differences between fee and non-fee cases? Social Work 5:46−52, 1960
5. Freud S: Further recommendations in the technique of psychoanalysis: On beginning the treatment, in Strachey J (ed): The Standard Edition of the Complete Works of Sigmund Freud (vol 12). London, Hogarth, 1958, pp 131−132
6. Menninger K: Theory of Psychoanalytic Technique, New York, Science Editions, 1961, p 32
7. Kubie L: Practical and Theoretical Aspects of Psychoanalysis. New York, Interanational Universities Press, 1950, p 136
8. Davids A: The relation of cognitive-dissonance theory to an aspect of psychotherapeutic practice. Am Psychol 19:329−332, 1964
9. Pope KS, Wilkinson L, Geller JD: National survey on psychotherapist attitudes toward fees. Paper presented to the annual meeting of the American Psychological Association, Montreal, 1980

10. Pope KS, Geller JD, Wilkinson L: Fee assessment and outpatient psychotherapy. J Consulting and Clinical Psychol 43:835–841, 1975
11. Balch P, Ireland JF, Lewis SB: Fees and therapy: Relation of source of payment to course of therapy at a community mental health center. J Consulting and Clinical Psychol 45:504, 1977
12. Brown R: Words and Things. Glencoe, The Free Press, 1958, p 93
13. Bourne LE, Ekstrand BR, Duminowski RL: The Psychology of Thinking. Englewood Cliffs, Prentice-Hall, 1971
14. Johnson DM: The Psychology of Thought and Judgment. New York, Harper & Row, 1955
15. Mischel W: Introduction to Personality. New York, Holt Rinehard and Winston, 1971
16. Seidman JM: The Adolescent. New York, Holt Rinehart and Winston, 1960
17. Skinner BF: The steep and thorny way to a science of behavior. Am Psychol 30:42–49, 1975
18. Kris E: On preconscious mental processes, in Rappaport D (ed): Organization and Pathology of Thought. New York, Columbia University Press, 1951, pp 474–493
19. Singer JL: Experimental studies of daydreaming and the stream of thought, in Pope K and Singer JL (eds): The Stream of Consciousness: Scientific Investigations into the Flow of Human Experience. New York, Plenum, 1978
20. Klinger E: Modes of normal conscious flow, in Pope KS and Singer J (eds): The Stream of Consciousness: Scientific Investigations into the Flow of Human Experience. New York, Plenum, 1978
21. Csikszentmihalyi M: Attention and the holistic approach to behavior, in Pope KS and Singer JL (eds): The Stream of Consciousness: Scientific Investigations into the Flow of Human Experience. New York, Plenum, 1978
22. Pope KS: How gender, solitude, and posture influence the stream of consciousness, in Pope KS and Singer JL (eds): The Stream in Consciousness: Scientific Investigations into the Flow of Human Experience. New York, Plenum Press, 1978
23. Pope KS and Singer JL: The Stream of Consciousness: Scientific Investigations into the Flow of Human Experience. New York, Plenum Press, 1978
24. Pope KS and Singer JL: Regulation of the stream of consciousness: Toward a theory of ongoing thought, in Schwartz GE and Shapiro D (eds): Consciousness and Self-Regulation: Advances in Research and Theory (vol 2). New York, Plenum Press, 1978
25. Pope KS, Levenson H, Schover L: Sexual intimacy in psychology training: Results and implications of a national survey. Am Psychol 34:682–689, 1979

PART IV

Complex and Ultimate Themes

Fritz Redlich

Introduction

If one were asked to describe three major changes in psychiatry during the last twenty-five years, one might suggest the following: First, there has been a modest upgrading from what Lewis Thomas calls a "no technology" field to "half-way technology." One aspect of such change is the development of basic neurobiology, which will eventually have great impact on psychiatric practice. Already some successful biological therapies have appeared, such as the treatments of bipolar affective psychosis with lithium, and schizophrenia with neuroleptic drugs (both discovered serendipitously). The second change is the development and acceptance of scientific thinking by psychiatrists. Today's well trained psychiatrist tries to employ scientific principles in his or her clinical endeavors with the same rigor as workers in other clinical specialties, even though such critical thinking often results initially in the recognition of one's ignorance. Third is the impact of professional ethics on the practice of medicine, including the practice of clinical psychiatry, and on psychiatric research. Ethical propositions, principles, and rules are pervasive in today's practice and research; for the first time, the rules are established not only by the expert-provider but by the consumer and his or her political, legal, or bureaucratic representatives.

The three articles in this section discuss the impact that psychiatric, psychological, and sociological research and humanistic scholarship in the field of ethics should have on the practice of clinical psychiatry. In point of fact, however, there is currently a lack of such research and scholarship which have impact on clinical psychiatry, and the articles examine this deficiency.

Richard Hough's article focuses most sharply on the problem. He recognizes that social and epidemiological research up to now have contributed little to the solution of clinical problems, because they have dealt with generalities and not with specific variables. Hough makes some concrete proposals for improving this. His model is derived from the Rahe-Arthur model dealing with the effects of life events on illness; with inadequate psychological and physiological mechanisms to deal with stress, the result is unsatisfactory coping and finally illness behavior. The Rahe-Arthur model is too broad and general, according to Hough, and he introduces more specific and complex variables: first, the socioeconomic characteristics of the stressed individual; second, types of stress factors; third, mediating responses, particularly varying perception of threats and the availability of adaptive resources, such as the existence of therapeutic facilities and social support and the individual's efficiency in using them; and fourth, different psychological outcomes depending on the interaction of these factors. In addition, he believes that the new diagnostic psychiatric taxonomy—DSM III—will permit researchers and clinicians to establish more specific relationships between sociocultural stresses and pathological outcomes. He illustrates this convincingly with hypothetical cases: e.g., why a clinical population of Mexican immigrant workers might be at risk to develop depressive disorders, and how the detailed scrutiny and understanding of the process might aid the clinician and public health worker to institute specific, meaningful interventions.

William Winslade calls attention to the fact that there has been very little empirical investigation of ethical behavior, not to speak of professional ethical behavior. This is not surprising, of course, as ethicists usually come from the tradition of philosophy and are trained in scholarly thinking, not in scientific research. Moritz Schlick, a philosopher of the Viennese School of Logical Positivism, said in one of his lectures that philosophers start where scientists end their endeavors. He illustrated this by drawing a picture of a mountain, the top enshrouded in clouds, the bottom clear. Scientists work at the bottom, philosophers in the clouds. Philosophers ask questions and rarely are able to give answers; scientists may give answers in the field of their expertise. Scientists have no answer to the question of ''what ought to be,'' but they can explore how ethical questions arise, how ethical decisions are made, and what ethical conflicts might be encountered.

Winslade proposes specifically to examine the rules which govern professional–client relationships and to investigate the impact on research of ethical and legal regulation by government and governing bodies. Such regulation has succeeded in protecting subjects, but it also has slowed down research and at times even stopped it altogether. Philosophers have discussed these issues from a utilitarian point of view (in terms of cost-benefit) and from a categorical point of view (in terms of what is right). A scientific approach to this problem would yield data, which could facilitate philosophical reflections and anchor them in facts. Investigating the behavior of researchers, subjects, and regulators (and the conflicts between them) would be of considerable benefit for current and future patients in clinical practice.

Winslade focuses on two major issues: how much discretion individual clinicians and researchers need in order to work effectively, and how governmental or bureaucratic regulation restricts such freedom or discretion. The pendulum has swung from an underprotection of the individual and patient, particularly members of disadvantaged populations (children, psychotic and retarded persons, and prisoners) to an undesirable overregulation and paternalism.

Norman Brill's article is a broad and intriguing essay about certain evils of our time and how modern psychiatry has deliberately or unwittingly gone along with them. He wrote his paper shortly after he returned from a short trip to China, where he was impressed with Chariman Mao's principle of serving the people and the obvious discipline of the Chinese masses. I had a similar experience in China, and I concur with many of Brill's views, but I am still unsure of the price such discipline exacts and what its consequences are.

Brill is very concerned about what he sees as a deterioration in society's mores in the West, and in part his article is a jeremiad on the decline of authority and discipline and the increase of selfishness in the "me society." But he recognizes that we live in a pluralistic society: though he questions the current minority demand for bilingual education, he would not deny them the right of free expression; though he wonders if some adults are constitutionally incapable of being parents (citing the opinion of Ashley Montagu), he realizes that licensed parenthood is absurd. In a society of complex and sometimes conflicting values, simplistic approaches will not help.

More specifically, Brill feels that modern psychiatry has lost sight of its primary concern of diagnosing, treating, and preventing major psychiatric disorders. He criticizes psychiatry for its overconcern with alleged societal causes of mental illness, such as poverty or racism. It is clear that psychiatric disorders occur among the wealthy and the poor alike, although there is increasing evidence that certain major disorders are more frequent among the poor and that lack of treatment—assuming that effective treatment exists—increases the plight of the impoverished mentally ill patient. In any case, it is important to understand that psychiatric problems are our primary concern and that poverty, ignorance, crime, and existential problems are secondary concerns. This may lead to a more strict definition of psychiatry as a medical specialty, as opposed to a universal science of man. This would result in a restriction of psychiatric activities—a painful but necessary job. This might become feasible if we as mental health professionals make an even more serious and committed effort to distinguish between facts and beliefs, between scientific knowledge and value judgments. This is difficult because much of what we do is not determined by the objective characteristics of a disorder or disease, but by social expectations of the sick role and the healer role. Even so, it is of the greatest importance to define core or primary tasks, and their boundaries. I believe this is important in all of medicine, but particularly in psychiatry.

The quest for scientific knowledge and its application to clinical practice will make this difficult task easier. It will also help if authors in psychiatry can identify their propositions as expert and scientific (with an operational approach), literary and philosophical, or as the commonsense statements of concerned citizens. While these are all necessary, they should not be confounded. A psychiatrist's task is not to solve the world's burning problems; it is to treat mental disorders based on the best available scientific evidence.

Norman Q. Brill

11
Psychosocial Determinants of Emotional Disorders

The effect that a culture can have on the incidence, diagnosis, and treatment of psychiatric disorders can be clearly demonstrated in a visit to the People's Republic of China.[1] This is not to say that all psychiatric disorders are of sociocultural origin. Many are secondary to organic disease of the brain (including disorders that are metabolic, toxic, infectious, degenerative, neoplastic, circulatory, allergic, etc.) and it is fairly well established that genetic and constitutional factors contribute to the development of nervous and mental disorders along with social, developmental and interpersonal stresses.

In China, some conditions (primarily character and behavior disorders) which in this country are regarded as illnesses are merely regarded as maladjustments. They require reeducation, socialization, and rehabilitation. In a country where essentially all are poor, and working to obtain the necessities of life, individuals are preoccupied with reality problems and relatively little attention is paid to persons with less severe psychopathology and neurotic (unrealistic) problems, especially since relatively little provision exists for dealing with them. Where all treatment is directed toward getting

Parts of this chapter are derived from Brill NQ: Preventive psychiatry. Psychiatr Opinion 14:30–34, 1977, by permission.

people back to work, where functional illness is regarded as a manifestation of preoccupation with self rather than with "service to the people," which is the China's slogan, there is little in the way of secondary gain.

Where there is some feeling that it is unpatriotic and antisocial to be disabled by an emotional disorder, it is understandable that psychiatric treatment does not have a very high priority as compared with other medical treatment. Gregorio Bermann reported that as late as 1965 there were no psychiatrists or psychologists who occupied themselves with delinquents, nor did he find any institutions for the retarded.[2] I believe this is still the case.

While there are clear and universally accepted concepts of the pathogenesis of most organic diseases, there is great variation in the importance attributed to specific stresses in the etiology of emotional illness from one culture to another. In China for example, lack of dedication to serving the people is regarded as playing a role in functional disorders, including schizophrenia and affective disorders, while in the United States in recent years, stresses such as poverty, racism and male chauvinism have been emphasized as prime factors in causing emotional illness. These differences in the understanding of emotional disorders obviously have great effect on how these disorders are treated, and beyond that, on theories and programs of prevention. In China, reeducation, rehabilitation, work, selflessness, and physical activity are emphasized and employed in treatment and prevention, while in the United States, the trend in recent years has focused on removal of stress and on catering to individual rights and needs. Life itself is characterized by stresses and since there is a relationship between stress and the incidence of emotional disorders, it is understandable that some behavioral scientists and clinicians would seek to eliminate as much stress as possible in the interest of the mental health of a population.

Others, who are inclined to believe that changing reality (that is, eliminating the stresses) is not only very difficult but at times impossible, try to focus on how people deal with stress and what there is about them that contributes to their inability to do so successfully. They try to help the person develop more effective methods of dealing with stress.

There is, however, a natural tendency to try to get rid of stress and how this is done depends in part on what is acceptable, possible and encouraged. Unemployment, for example, is a stress. In a society like China, there is no unemployment. In our society, there are people who are able to work but don't—not because there are no jobs but because they elect not to take the jobs that are available. If they were not taken care of by others who do work, there would undoubtedly be less unemployment. So the way that people deal with stress is to some degree orchestrated by the society.

Poverty is another stress, but a more complicated one. Poverty in some places is defined by survival levels and in other places by comfort levels. Additionally, the poor in any society constitute an extremely heterogeneous group.

In China, where survival is at stake, the solution is for everyone to work as much as they can, with the rewards geared to the person's effort and productivity, not to needs. In this respect China is not truly communistic. In the United States, which professes to be a capitalistic society, we are concerned with needs. It partly explaine why every program that has been designed to eliminate poverty has failed. We cater to poverty and not to what is needed to eliminate it.

The currently popular belief, that mental illness can in great part be prevented by eliminating poverty, racism, and inequality of the sexes, is unfortunately a mistaken notion that is somewhat remindful of the premature application of partial knowledge that stemmed from Freud's observation that repression of hostile and sexual impulses in childhood and conflict contributed to the development of emotional disorders later in life. The solution to some educators and mental health professionals was to encourage rearing children who would be free of conflict and repression. They encouraged free expression of sexual and hostile feelings, exposure of children to sex as a natural phenomenon and, as a consequence, instead of sexual neuroses, some of these children developed character and behavior disorders. They acted out their feelings and impulses, often showed crude and uninhibited behavior that offended others, and stimulated either rejection or retaliation, and they could not understand why they weren't happy. Now encounter sessions and marathons, which may be derivatives of this same approach, encourage people to overcome their reluctance to vent their anger, and other feelings, on others.

It is already possible to see some of the negative derivatives of the emphasis on removing social stresses as the main thrust of preventive mental health programs. When efforts were made to get the California Department of Health to improve the staffing and treatment programs of the State Hospital, the Director of Health, believing that mental illness was the result of social evils, made no distinction between human suffering (that required social action) and mental illness (that required treatment) and therefore did nothing to improve conditions in the hospitals. In this connection, it is interesting that the Joint Commission on Mental Health in Children would claim that racism is the number one mental health problem facing the nation today.

It is true that community studies have shown a higher incidence of mental illness in lower social classes, and there is no question that poverty is often associated with excessive family stress, undernourishment, poor physical health and negative attitudes toward life. Exposure to racial prejudice is certainly not conducive to a positive outlook. But psychiatric disorders are the result of forces that go beyond these stresses and it is obvious that all persons who are poor or exposed to racial prejudice are not ill.

It is as unscientific to say that poverty breeds mental illness as it is to say that wealth prevents it. Those who have worked intensively with psychiatric patients have had the opportunity to see how much interpersonal friction, unhappiness and conflict exist within families that are not underprivileged, and to observe the divorces, alcoholism, drug abuse, depressions, psychosomatic disorders, neuroses and psychoses that result.

There are still vast differences of opinion among sociologists concerning the magnitude of the roles played in the development of mental disorders by low socioeconomic status or other concomitant variables of poverty. While ecological studies have clearly shown that incidence rates for mental disorders in the United States are highest in areas populated by groups of low socioeconomic status, it has not yet been clearly established whether this is the result of excessive stress (direct or intrafamilial) of the poverty condition or of downward drifting of mentally disturbed persons. Also, it is interesting that in reviewing the dynamic formulations of patients' illness contained in hospital chart summaries, I found that poverty was rarely, if ever, mentioned as a cause.

We cannot ignore what has become increasingly obvious in the past fifty years—the importance of early childhood experiences in the emotional development of an individual. What the child, with its unique genetic make-up and personality characteristics that are present from birth, is exposed to in its family is a crucial determinant of its later adult adjustment and behavior. The role of the mother is primary and the nature of her interaction with her infant cannot be ignored or minimized. The father, too, is important but in early life he still generally occupies a secondary role.

Ross and Glaser studied a group of Black and Mexican-American males from seriously disadvantaged backgrounds to determine what factors differentiated those who were able to "make it" (i.e., were well and functioning in society without public assistance or intervention) from those who could not (i.e., were unemployed, living in poverty areas, and in need of assistance).[3] The successful ones had at least one strong parent (or parent surrogate like a grandmother) who had high expectations of the child and provided sustained loving care and constant discipline. Their childhood time was described as warm. They participated in school activities and never received failing grades in school. They had positive attitudes toward themselves, felt pride in accomplishment, gained some recognition, and were fully supporting their own families, if married; their marriage was cohesive, with positive feelings towards their wives. Their parents encouraged them to speak proper English, and emphasized religious values at home. They believed that hard work and education were the best means of getting ahead and never had trouble with the law.

The unsuccessful ones tended to have no caring person in their families who presented clear standards or had high expectations for them. The home atmosphere was apt to be neutral or hostile. They did not participate in school activities; parental discipline was inconsistent; they occasionally or frequently received failing grades, had negative attitudes about themselves, never felt pride in accomplishment and never felt successful; they were not fully supporting their present families, were uninvolved in their marriage or estranged; had negative feelings toward their wives and tended to be separated or divorced. Their parents were not concerned with the way they expressed themselves and did not stress religious values. The typical unsuccessful one looks upon hustling as a good way to get ahead or else doesn't know how to do it. He has had trouble with the law both as a juvenile and as an adult. (He was charged with delinquency as a juvenile and with criminal offense as an adult.)

Their present situations tend to be expressions of a general life style that appears to be strongly related to the attitudes of their parents; the expectations that parents had for them and the demands that they made of them. In the black families, the more effective parent was the mother. In the Mexican-American families, success was more dependent on the presence of an effective father.[3]

What this suggests and needs to be faced, if we are really serious and realistic about preventing emotional disorders, is that there are many parents who are incapable of rearing mentally healthy children as a consequence of their own emotional, intellectual or characterological difficulties.

Ashley Montagu, an anthropologist who has long been an observer of the human scene, points out, "It has been said that man is the only 150 lb. nonlinear servomechanism that can be wholly reproduced by unskilled labor." Further, he says that ". . . the capacity to reproduce is something that must be at least as much subject to control as taking the life of another individual. While there are sanctions against murder, there are no sanctions against people bringing children into the world for whom they are unable to care. The murderer usually takes the life of one person. The irresponsible proliferator throws away the lives of many persons and saddles them upon a society and upon a world that are unable to meet their needs as human beings, (so that) in consequence they suffer disastrously from the presence of so many superfluous people." He claims that "no one should be permitted to have children unless clear evidence of his or her ability to serve as an adequate parent can be given—as people now have to do to be able to drive a car or build a house."[4]

While I do not endorse the proposal to license parents, if social psychiatrists are serious about preventing mental and emotional illness, they are going to have to consider in any preventive program the powerful effect that parents have on their children and the extent to which emotional disorders are rooted in early childhood experiences. There is a suggestion that some mental health workers entertain the myth that if people are to be mentally healthy, there should be no unhappiness, no anxiety, no conflict, no struggle, no emotional discomfort, and possibly no unsatisfied need, and that if any of these exist, it is because of some defect in society. At a White House briefing on crime, social agency representatives implied that society is at fault when an individual commits a crime because society did not recognize and meet his or her needs, and that therefore no one should be locked up. Emphasis has shifted from helping individuals adjust to society to having society adjust to individuals, and social reform has to be justified on the basis of health reasons rather than for ethical, humanitarian or political reasons.

Poverty or prejudice now must be eliminated, it is said, not for ethical or humanitarian reasons, but because they are bad for mental health. In order to permit women to take time off with pay during pregnancy, pregnancy had to be regarded as a disability, putting it in the category of illness rather than a natural biologic event.

An example of society adjusting to individuals, rather than expecting individuals to adjust to society, is the recent ruling in California that instruction in elementary schools will have to be given in Spanish as well as in English, and election ballots must be printed in both English and Spanish. While the reasons for this are obvious, it is a far cry from the expectation years ago—when there were mass immigrations of Irish, German, Scandinavians, Italians, and Jews to the country—that immigrants had the responsibility to learn the language of the country to which they had come.

I mention these things because they are currently regarded by many as steps in the right direction toward eliminating mental illness and emotional discomfort. There are many other, perhaps even more important, social stresses that need relief: unemployment, inadequate housing, malnutrition, lack of transportation, insufficient recreational facilities, inadequate legal assistance, lack of clothing, increasing crime, and violence, and even polluted air and water. Are these to be eliminated just because they are bad for mental health and will mental illness disappear if all these are eliminated? The desire to help pregnant women who are self-supporting, and the urge to make life easier for Mexican-American children who are in our schools are understandable, but one may wonder if gratifying insatiable demands and catering to infinite expectations are, in the long run, going to advance the mental health of our nation.

There has been a dramatic increase in the number of psychiatrists and mental health workers of all kinds over the past 25 years, and impressive social advances have been made to provide economic benefits through social security, unemployment insurance, aid to dependent children, medical care, better nutrition through food stamps and school meals, social equality, equal opportunity, civil rights, etc. These have not been accompanied by a visible decrease in mental illness, crime, human unhappiness, or world tension, all of which seem to be getting worse.

We tend to believe that something approaching a utopia is possible through technological advances. Yet every technological advance in the history of human kind has brought problems in its wake. Theoretically, a society protected from stress might end up being more vulnerable to stress, since every spectrum of life from birth to death is accompanied by stress. Jonas Salk, when asked if the infectious disease model that involved a pathogenic agent, transmission and host resistance could be applied to mental illness, said it could not. He explained that when an organism was injected with an excessive dose of antigen, it developed an antibody paralysis; that is, it did not produce any protecting antibodies. If infants or young children were exposed to too much stress at a time when they were too young and their ego defenses were not sufficiently developed, he wondered if a similar paralysis would prevent them from generating the type and amount of defenses that are required for normal emotional development. If there is any validity to this comparison, the need to ensure the proper rearing of children becomes paramount in any preventive psychiatry program.

One essential in the rearing of children would be to inculcate them with the expectation that they will be required as adults to be responsible for themselves. One can predict that a society that is reared on the principle of its rights, without mention of its responsibilities, will never be a mentally healthy society. I wonder if the current trend of expecting the government to cater to every individual's desires, and encouraging people to believe this is their right, is stimulating a massive regression of our society to an oral dependent state from which there may be no recovery without a radical, painful change in the entire sociopolitical system.

Our culture surrounds us like the air and most of the time we are quite unaware of it. A culture consists of the total of all the rules, attitudes, customs, expectations, and requirements of a society, just as the personality of an individual (which is different from all others) consists of the sum total of that person's expectations, manners, behavior, emotional reactions, and method of dealing with life and others.

As a consequence of the tremendous increase in population that has increased the density of living, the increase in mobility and communication, the greater sophistication of the public that is associated with increased political activity, the increase in the standard of living and degrees of affluence, along with a much greater degree of interdependence, the culture of the United States is clearly quite different today from what it was 200 years ago (and even from what it was 50 years ago). Considering just the attitudes toward behavior, dress, religion and work, the change is very obvious. Minor breeches of behavior were punished. There was little tolerance for deviation from accepted norms. The early Americans struggled against a harsh reality and had few others than themselves and close neighbors to rely on. They lived or died in great part as a consequence of their own efforts.

How different expectations and attitudes and behavior are today. Instead of wanting more children, who were highly valued and regarded as assets when the country was primarily agrarian, an increasing fraction of our people either wants no children or regards them as burdens or unwelcome responsibilities. No longer are they assets, but contributors to people pollution and overpopulation. There is an expectation that it is up to the government to take care of its population from birth to death—to ensure that people are provided with education, medical services, adequate income, food, shelter, and protection not just from enemies but from each other. With consumer protective agencies, now it is the seller who must beware and not the buyer. If anything untoward happens to a person, there is a pervading attitude that it is someone else's fault or someone else's responsibility to make amends. "The University of Michigan has recently been sued by a former student for $838,000.00 for the mental anguish he suffered after being given a 'D' grade in a German course—where he expected an 'A'. A prisoner who escaped from a county jail in Pennsylvania and was recaptured and had to serve extra time, sued the sheriff and two guards for $1,000,000.00 for letting him escape. Two football fans, claiming that an official had made a call that resulted in their team's loss, sued because they had been robbed of their right to see a victory . . . Recently a man filed a million dollar suit against the Coors Beer Company because he "pickled his brain by drinking large amounts of 3.2% beer that he didn't know was intoxicating." According to a former president of the American Bar Association, "The concept of individual responsibility has been seriously eroded. Today, people expect to be protected even from their own gullibility."[5]

Landau comments about the unwholesome perspective of our society and relates that people jumped into a wrecked suburban train so they could walk off and claim injury, and that people have sued the owners of a ski slide when they have broken limbs coming down.[6]

If they are unhappy or unsuccessful, they prefer to think it's their parents' fault, or because they were disadvantaged by racism, poverty, or male chauvinism.

It is not unusual to see the attitude that it is the criminal who needs protection from society, not society from the criminal; or that it is the criminal's rights that need defending, not society's.

The increased dependence and reliance on government and others has been associated with an increase in concern about self—what has been called "Narcissistic Generation" or the *Me* Generation—that is characterized by preoccupation with one's own pleasures, safety, and advancement, and a "Hell with the Public" attitude. It has been associated with increases in divorce, crime, emotional tension, anxiety, job dissatisfaction, conflict, lower birth rate, and changes in standards of sexual behavior, language, dress, and work.

Lasch, in "The Culture of Narcissism," alludes to the preoccupation with self and pursuit of happiness that characterizes American culture today.[7] "A once rugged and resourceful America is now seething with a destructive oedipal rage masquerading as the pleasure principle." "Having overthrown feudalism and slavery and then outgrown its own personal and familial form, capitalism has evolved a new political ideology, welfare liberalism, which absolves individuals of moral responsibility and treats them as victims of social circumstance. It has evolved new modes of social control which deal with the deviant as a patient and substitute medical rehabilitation for punishment. It has given rise to a new culture, the Narcissistic Culture of our time." He proves his claim by pointing to the change in greetings from "Goodbye" (short for "God be with you") to "Have a nice day, enjoy!"

According to Andrew Hacker,[8] "More people seem studiously absorbed in themselves than at any time in our history. More is involved than simple selfishness. Individuals place a high estimate on their own importance. One casualty has been the American marriage." He asks, "How can two so preoccupied creatures share space with one another?" He reminds us that a long time ago de Tocqueville, who commented on the American culture and character, observed that inhabitants of democratic countries are haunted by a strange melancholy in the midst of their abundance. It is more apparent now. Hacker suggests that this self-preoccupation may be the consequence of our efficient production (and affluence) that gives rise to more leisure time in which to be preoccupied with self. It explains the appearance of bumper stickers that say, "If it feels good, do it," and books like, "Winning Through Intimidation," and "Looking Out for Number One."

Young people are increasingly reluctant to make the kind of commitment to each other that is implied in a marriage. They want to get out easily when they no longer enjoy each other, and be free of any obligation. They maintain that society has no right to prescribe how they should behave (sexually and otherwise), dress, speak, or work as long as they don't hurt anyone else. They should be free to drug themselves into a state of perpetual euphoria or stupor if they wish—and they don't regard having to be taken care of by the rest of society, when they can no longer function, as hurting anyone else.

As pointed out by Jones, trust in all types of institutions, but especially government, has declined.[9] "People are more prosperous today; they live longer than they did 50 years ago, yet life's rewards still fall short of expectations—whatever the cause. Many Americans doubt the strength and even the validity of old values and are skeptical about the quality of their lives in a disruptive age of technology." Jones sees a quest for belief in the rise in "old time religion" and seems to agree that "a radical departure from the open-ended values evident today in such things as easy divorces and the emphasis on pleasure" is required along with a commitment that goes beyond self interest, if belief is to be reborn. He also refers to Karl Menninger's book "Whatever Became of Sin?", in which it is pointed out how "sins" have become "crimes" and, finally, "symptoms" that are treated as "illness" which then is blamed on anyone or anything except the person himself. Jones quotes Menninger who maintains "A conscious sense of guilt and implicit or explicit repentance would be consequences of an acknowledgement of error, transgression, offense and responsibility—in short, sin. This might revive the idea of personal responsibility and possibly turn the tide of our aggressions and of the moral struggle, in which much of the world population is engaged."

Marvin Stone, respected editor of the U.S. News World Report,[10] asks in the same vein, "What kind of people are we?". He refers to how we "shrug off almost everything now, moving on—with a lot of help from the omnivorous media—to the next fleeting titillation . . . It's as if we are beyond making distinctions, beyond caring . . . Third graders are selling dope, White House aides are buying it. Our appetite for violence is insatiable . . . The ennui of affluence can overwhelm a nation." In this condition, nothing seems to call for striving or to demand common effort. He writes, "Certainly we have the intelligence to understand that we are going through one more social revolution in this country, and the challenge is to preserve the best of the past and embrace the good in the new. But it will take leadership to define and inspire a common purpose, and desire by the rest of us to pursue it." I wonder if he realizes how much of what he says resembles what Chairman Mao said in China. President Carter, in his January 1979 State of the Union Address, admits that the problems we face today are different from those that confronted earlier generations of Americans. They are more subtle and more complex and few of them can be solved by government alone.

Army regulations in the past differentiated between illness that was secondary to an individual's misconduct and that which was not. The differences have now become almost obliterated and again society has assumed the responsibility for what a person does to himself. A person doesn't have to work to receive welfare or other aid if he doesn't like the job that is offered him. A person who commits a serious crime can successfully plea bargain and get off with a lesser or no punishment because the courts are overburdened and the prisons incapable of handling the large number who would otherwise be incarcerated. People are dependent on thousands of others they don't know (and who live in unknown distant places) for their food, energy sources for heat and light, transportation, garbage collection, protection, etc., and are powerless to defend themselves against the demands of special interest groups.

With all of these increases in dependency on government and on others and with a diminution in the rules which govern the orderly functioning of a society, we are witnessing an increase in cults, unhappiness, depression, anxiety, dissatisfaction, conflict, divorce, demonstrations, disobedience, arson, vandalism, rape, mugging, robberies—all of which have some significance for psychiatry.

How people deal with stress and reality depends in part on what is acceptable, possible, or encouraged. The culture of a society can have a great effect on the way basic instincts are expressed and on the incidence of many of the emotional disorders we are not only called upon to treat but to prevent. Freud said that work is the chief means of binding an individual to reality. Thomas Sowell, a black economist at UCLA, in his book "Race and Economics," points out that the greatest dilemma in attempts to raise ethnic minority income is that those methods which have historically proved successful—self-reliance, work skills, education and business experience—are all slow developing, while the methods which are more direct and immediate—job quotas, charity, subsidies and preferential treatment—tend to undermine self-reliance and pride of achievement in the long run. He feels that jobs are a first and indispensable necessity.[11]

The solution of the many distressing problems of society, which are related to mental health, will involve a resolution of the conflict over whether primary concern should be focused on the individual's freedom to do as he or she wishes, or on what is best for society as a whole.

It seems clear that a preventive psychiatry that focuses entirely on eliminating all stress and on gratifying human desires is bound to fail. While we must strive to improve the quality of life for all, we cannot lose sight of the fact that man is a social animal who must, in the course of his development, learn to tolerate the frustration, anxiety, conflict, disappointment and irrationality that inevitably is part of everyone's life. Society should not be allowed to be misled by those who, for political reasons or because they are trying to recreate their own childhoods as they were or should have been, stimulate expectations of utopia that leads to inevitable and massive disappointments. Donald Campbell, President of the American Psychological Association, in his address to that body chided his fellow psychologists for siding with self-gratification over self-restraint and for regarding guilt as a neurotic symptom. He believes that "there is a biological bias in favor of self-seeking, uninhibited behavior" and that "to counter this bias, human societies have evolved strong ethical and religious rules favoring the group over the individual." According to Campbell, "all of the modern psychologies are individualistically hedonistic, explaining all human behavior in terms of individual pleasure and pain, individual needs and drives . . . They not only describe man as selfishly motivated but 'implicitly or explicitly' teach that he ought to be so."[12] In her address to the American Psychiatric Association in May 1975, Margaret Mead criticized psychiatrists who have done little to protect children from emotional damage and abuse, although they know a great deal about broken homes and their effects on children. Society is in an exceedingly dangerous period, she pointed out. "The profession may be placing too much emphasis on social consciousness . . . it might better attempt to bring out the best in people, like that brought out in time of war: their sacrifice, loyalty, and unselfishness."[13]

And more recently Douglas McLean, in his presidential address to the Canadian Psychiatric Association, said, "Health, security and creature comforts may well be goals to seek, but to suggest that they are inherent and basic human rights is wrong. It is wrong because it carries with it the implication that man has the right to freedom from all discomfort at all times, and this is the message that bombards us incessantly, not only in the political process but in the educational and marketing process (TV commercials)." He added, "Now having exhausted the field of economic and social security, politicians have been casting about trying to find new ways to defend our rights and they have found a fertile field in the realm of civil rights. In a recent address to the American Bar Association, Solzhenitsyn stated that 'The defense of individual rights has reached such extremes as to make society as a whole defenseless against certain individuals.' It took a man who fled from a communist dictatorship to tell us that it is time in the West to defend not so much human rights as human obligations."[14]

One thing is clear. Nothing (including society and its government) remains the same. Change is inevitable and we are experiencing it now in an accelerated form. The change comes about in an attempt to deal with population stresses, and it also generates its own stresses. Each political system is characterized by its own stresses and will be burdened with emotional disorders that may vary in their manifestations and their response to remedial measures. People being what they are will always have problems and will always create problems. One thing is certain, we are a long way off from solving the problems, resolving the conflicts and preventing their negative consequences.

REFERENCES

1. Brill NQ: Preventive psychiatry. Psychiatr. Opinion 14:30–34, 1977
2. Bermann G: Mental health in China, in Kiev A (ed): Psychiatry in the Communist World. New York, Science House, 1968

3. Ross HL, Glaser EM: Making it out of the ghetto. Professional Psychol 4:347–356, 1973

4. Montagu A: Second thoughts. Hum Behav 4:10, 1975

5. Why everybody is suing everybody. U.S. News & World Report, Dec. 4, 1978, p 50

6. Landau RL:What you should know about estrogens. J Am Med Assoc 241:51, 1979

7. Why everybody is suing everybody. Time (Special Report), Jan. 8, 1979, p 76

8. Hacker A: Firing at Narcissus from a barricade of books. Wall Street Journal (editorial), Jan. 26, 1979

9. Jones GE: "The doubting America"—A growing breed. U.S. News & World Report, Feb. 26, 1979, pp 74–75

10. Stone M: What kind of people are we? U.S. News & World Report (editorial), Feb. 5, 1979, p 88

11. Sowell T: Race and Economics. New York, David McKay, 1975

12. Campbell DT: Morals make a comeback. Time, Sept. 15, 1975, p 94

13. Mead M: Dr. Mead suggests nonprofessionals as patients' listening posts. Clin Psychiatr News 3(7):9, 1975

14. McLean D: CPA president sees risk in upward mobility. Psychiatr News, Jan. 19, 1979, p 21

Richard L. Hough

12

Socio-Cultural Issues in Research and Clinical Practice: Closing the Gap

The problem of deriving clinical prevention, intervention, and postvention treatment programs from socio-cultural studies of psychological disorder has long plagued health service delivery policy makers. This chapter is written out of concern and acknowledgement that a considerable gap does in fact exist between such research and clinical practice. The author will contend that the historical development and methodological limitations of this field have precluded much specific clinically relevant research and prevented more mutually enhancing interface between research and practice. Moreover, the author will argue that the lack of a multifaceted etiological model of socio-cultural impacts on psychiatric impairment and the lack of an intervention implication assessment paradigm have impeded the communication between researchers and clinicians, and will supply such an etiological model and assessment paradigm. Finally, research results within a particular subsection of the overall field of psychiatric epidemiology will be presented and discussed in relation to the proposed assessment paradigm. The author thus hopes to demonstrate that the gap between research and clinical practice can be closed, at least along certain seams, and that the stitching together may be less of a chore than might be imagined.

Before these goals can be pursued, however, a caveat must be introduced. The reader should be aware that the author is not presuming to be able to provide a complete overview of the clinical implications of any and all research casting light on the linkages between socio-cultural factors and psychological disorder. Instead, the author will limit his focus to that socio-cultural research tradition in which he has been most intimately and directly involved—the field survey of psychiatric impairment in general populations with particular emphasis on linkages between such impairment and life change. Direct extrapolations from the findings and practical implications of this research tradition to others may not be appropriate. However, the author assumes that the problem of derivation of treatment implications from research would be considered significant by virtually any researcher or clinician interested in the impact of an individual's socio-cultural environment on his or her physical and mental health.

ORIGINS OF THE GAP BETWEEN PSYCHIATRIC EPIDEMIOLOGICAL RESEARCH AND CLINICAL PRACTICE

At first blush, it would seem that psychiatric epidemiology should have produced information of immediate and specific use to clinicians. Generally speaking, the research is carried out by investigators who are cognizant of and often involved in clinical work. The areas under systematic investigation— identifying high risk populations and testing etiological models—would also appear to have significant and immediate implications for health care efforts. However, several factors have precluded the development of research findings with specific, usable clinical relevance.

The first, and perhaps the most significant problem, has been that of developing a capability to reliably measure psychiatric impairment in field survey research. To be sure, knowledge of the epidemiology of psychiatric disorder has increased greatly since the pioneering work of Faris and Dunham in the 1930's.[1] Following World War II particularly, a number of researchers began to address the issue of the prevalence of psychiatric impairment in communities. The methodological vehicles for these studies were symptoms scales—lists of symptoms experienced with items summed to provide total psychiatric impairment scale scores.[2-4] The symptoms scales used in these studies presumably measured the likelihood of "caseness," and the validity of the measures were determined by prediction of hospitalization. The advantages of this method included avoiding problems with the unreliability of psychiatric diagnosis, allowing estimation of community prevalence of mental disorders based on careful sampling techniques, and providing data linking a wide variety of social structural, role, and psychological variables to mental health.

The major disadvantage of these studies was that they failed to specify the relationship between a scale value of mental impairment and any specific, diagnosable disease. Clinical implications of findings thus became difficult to identify and understand. For example, the best that could be derived as "practical" prevention or intervention efforts from the research might have been a program for screening segments of the population identified as high risk for specific diagnosable impairment, but to even begin to design such a treatment program, the type and rates of impairment have to be established. A program contingent upon screening, say, all lower class populations in the country for diagnosably significant levels of depression based on the research finding that there is an inverse relationship between social class and depression, would constitute a tremendously expensive and inefficient form of intervention. Moreover, the information generated would be of little direct use to clinical practitioners operating within institutional settings. Knowledge of the brute fact that lower class clients have a higher propensity for some unspecific form of impairment is not particularly helpful in identifying the most appropriate treatment regimen and institutional health service delivery program.

Closing the gap between large scale psychiatric epidemiological survey research and clinical practice has not only been hampered by the inability of researchers to develop diagnostically sensitive survey instruments to assess psychiatric impairment, but stitching this seam together has also been complicated by several problems with the instrumentation, such as:

1. Focusing only on a limited number of psychological, psychophysiological, and physical symptoms, thereby excluding other salient indicators of impairment (such as antisocial behaviors) and underemphasizing severe symptoms, both necessary considerations for meaningful clinical assessment;
2. Providing only unidimensional measures of impairment which ignore critical distinctions between types of mental disorders which have qualitatively different expressions (in symptomatology, etiology, prognosis and treatment outcome) and which are likely to demonstrate differential patterns of relationships with social epidemiological variables;
3. Concentrating on the prevalence of specific symptoms with insufficient regard for chronicity and recurrence of symptoms, which may be important for assessment of current psychiatric conditions (i.e., personality disorders or bipolar affective disorders);
4. Not distinguishing between primary and secondary impairment, a crucial distinction for clinical treatment.

It should be pointed out that not *all* the problems have stemmed from the difficulties of survey researchers in developing relevant, reliable measures of impairment appropriate to their technology and field conditions. On the clinical side, such additional difficulties have been encountered as:

1. Inadequately defined psychiatric diagnostic categories disallowing operationalization as research instruments (i.e., with objective inclusion and exclusion criteria);
2. Generally highly unreliable clinical diagnoses which are consequently difficult to utilize in research;
3. Clinical judgements of psychiatric impairment and diagnosis which are themselves subject to questions of validity and thus do not provide an absolute criterion on which to validate measures of psychiatric impairment.

In recent years, several groups of investigators have attempted to overcome some of these limitations in developing measures of psychiatric impairment that are both clinically relevant and useful as research tools. An interview schedule (PERI) containing a number of scales reflecting homogeneous groupings of symptoms has been developed by Dohrenwend at the Social Psychiatry Research Unit at Columbia.[5] But perhaps even more crucially, parallel development of interviewing techniques modeled closely on clinical diagnostic refinements specifying behavioral inclusion and exclusion criteria for various diagnostic categories is currently underway and gaining increased support.[6-10] The Schedule for Affective Disorders and Schizophrenia – Lifetime Version (SADS-L) interview is composed of questions concerning current symptoms, lifetime episodes of psychiatric disturbance, and clinical aspects of current episodes of illness at peak severity.[11] The order and progression of the questions have been designed to systematically rule in and rule out explicit diagnoses defined by the Research Diagnostic Criteria (RDC) developed by Spitzer.[9] The Renard Interview Schedule (RIS) developed by Robins and her associates is a similar but more highly structured diagnostic interview based on the Feighner diagnostic criteria.[10,12] The Diagnostic Interview Schedule (DIS) is currently being developed by Robins and advantageously combines the SADS-L and the RIS with a broader range of psychiatric diagnoses corresponding to the categories and criteria of the American Psychiatric Association's DSM-III as well as with more highly specified levels of severity. These advancements in the specification and standardization of diagnostic criteria and interviewing techniques have greatly reduced sources of unreliability in psychiatric diagnosis and exhibit more potential for generating more clinically relevant information in field studies than the previous symptoms checklist approach.

Nevertheless, it is not argued here that simply generating information concerning the incidence and prevalence of clinically relevant forms of psychiatric impairment will, in and of itself, close the gap between psychiatric epidemiology and psychiatric practice. Clearly, there are many origins of the gap which are not directly related to the measurement problem. For example, there is a tendency for researchers to be more concerned with addressing basic research issues in their specialized fields of research than with clinical application of their findings and a corresponding tendency for clinicians to become so involved in the day-to-day contingencies and problems of health service delivery, career pressures, and bureaucratic/administrative demands that they do not have the time to read, absorb, interpret, and relevantly integrate research findings into their practices. There is no way these factors will disappear in the foreseeable future, and in fact, one would not want to see a complete amalgamation of the two, since in order to continue to make their unique contributions, research and clinical practice should remain fairly discrete and distinct.

However, at least two new possible developments in socio-cultural epidemiology and etiology of psychological disorder, in addition to improved measurement, promise to facilitate communication. These are the construction of (1) a general etiological model of social-cultural factors affecting illness behavior, and (2) a paradigm for the assessment of the clinical relevance of research findings. Preliminary suggestions for such a model (Fig. 12−2) and paradigm (Fig. 12−3) are presented below, along with an attempt to demonstrate some of their possible clinical applications from life change and psychiatric impairment research findings.

A NEW MODEL OF MAJOR SOCIO-CULTURAL VARIABLE AND IMPAIRMENT OUTCOME LINKAGES

The most often employed and well known theoretical conceptualization of the relationship between stressful life events, life change, and illness is the Rahe-Arthur model summarized in Figure 12−1.[13,14] Stemming directly from the research tradition of Hinkle and Wolff,[15] this model suggests that past experiences in a person's life can impinge on the individual and provoke some alteration in his or her normal life functioning patterns. This shift in the

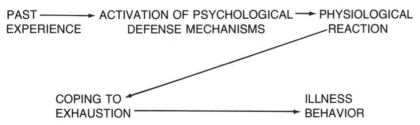

Fig. 12−1. The Rahe-Arthur theoretical model for life event effects on illness. (Adapted from Rahe RH, Arthur RJ: Life change and illness studies. J Human Stress 4:3−15, 1978)

established behavioral equilibrium, in turn, activates psychological defenses and coping strategies. Presumably, when the defenses and coping behaviors prove insufficient to deal positively with the amount of change required of the individual, illness behavior results.

The Rahe-Arthur model reflects a prototypical psychiatric-medical conceptualization of how an individual's social setting and past experience might act in relation to the onset of psychiatric illness. In this model, the total impact of social environment tends to be perceived as a simple, undifferentiated stimulus which, together with genetic and biological causal agents, produces undifferentiated psychiatric (or other) illness behavior.

By contrast, the proposed "Model of Major Socio-Cultural Variable and Impairment Outcome Linkages" depicted in Figure 12–2 suggests that the potential richness of knowledge to be gained from studying the impact of socio-environmental variables on psychiatric impairment cannot be appreciated until theoretical constructs become more complex and differentiated. Thus, Figure 12–2 represents an attempt to synthesize a number of variables which are typically involved and investigated in current life events research.

Note that virtually all of the elements under the new rubrics of socio-economic characteristics, stressors, and mediators are subsumed under the single, general designation of "past experience" in the old Rahe-Arthur model. By specifying and elaborating on particular elements as factors, it is clear that a more complicated model develops quickly from a relatively simplistic one. Notice also that the specific outcome variable of "psychiatric impairment" is also itself differentiated in the new model into the various major *types* of impairment. This reflects a growing emphasis in the field of stress research with which the author is acquainted: to generate theoretical etiological models which may explain variations in general populations of the incidence and prevalence of specific types of psychiatric impairment. This approach is based on the notion that interacting sets of variable elements in an individual's past experience which may have produced one specific outcome, such as depression, in that individual, may differ considerably from the sets of variable elements which may have produced another specific outcome in another individual, such as schizophrenia.

Besides detailing the variable elements involved in a person's past experience and breaking down compound categories into their logical components, the model proposed in Figure 12–2 is more complex in other ways.

Cumulative, multi-leveled, interactional, and reciprocal relationships between socio-economic characteristics, stressors, mediators, and impairment outcomes are visualized as opposed to disintricate, unidirectional effects. The age and sex of an individual, for example, may interact with marital stressors, both in terms of life change and life strain, to heighten the perceived threat of retirement while the absence of adaptive resources and/or the presence of

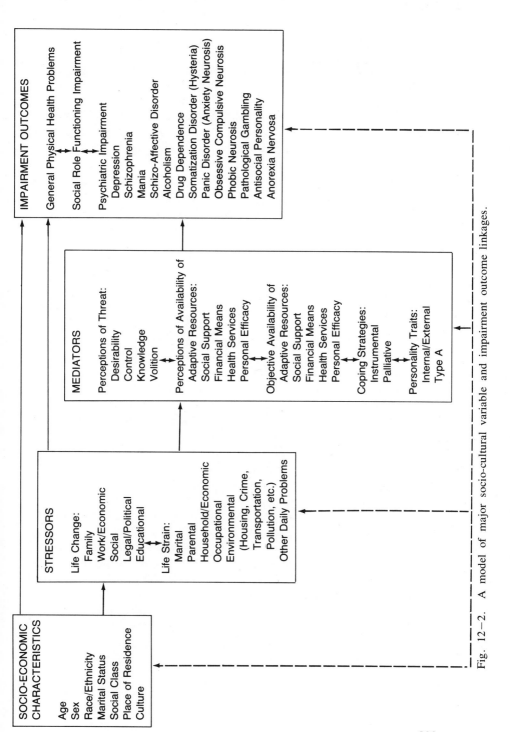

Fig. 12–2. A model of major socio-cultural variable and impairment outcome linkages.

particular coping styles and personality traits may interact with age, sex, and marital stressors to produce a depressive disorder in response to the individual's retirement.

Further, a "boomerang" effect between the compound categories (feedback indicated by the dotted lines) suggests that psychiatric impairment in the form of a major depressive disorder, for example, may impact negatively back onto the individual's ability to maintain given social class position responsibilities, onto the degree of stress and strain present in the individual's household, onto his or her tendency to perceive stressors as threatening, and/or onto his or her ability to mobilize social support or other adaptive resources, thus possibly generating additional or new (and probably more severe) impairment.

The critical suggestion is, then, that a more complex theoretical model may have the advantage of sensitizing the researcher/clinician to a broad range of factors which may, as a consequence of their interactional, transactional, reciprocal, and/or cumulative effects produce a particular form of health impairment. The new model is not intended to be directly amenable to rigorous statistical testing, but aspires to portray an overarching organization, in breadth and in depth, of a range of variables which might have considerable heuristic value in developing clinically relevant interpretations of research findings. If a particular research finding can be integrated into a general model of relationships between socio-cultural variables and impairment outcomes, its appropriateness as a nodal point of potential clinical intervention efforts can begin to be assessed in comparison to other possible nodal points.

For example, let us suppose that research demonstrates that a particular set of sex, age, racial, marital status and social class individuals (e.g., male, older, minority, single, lower class) is especially vulnerable to the constellation of stressors surrounding retirement, but that the same constellation of stressors is relatively benign for the same set of individuals when the intensity of life strains and negative perceptions of retirement as threatening are weak or absent. The appropriate health servicing response might then be to set up a clinical prevention program aimed at modifying negative perceptions of retirement in occupations disproportionately occupied by that particular set of individuals. Or, should family support mechanisms be proved by research to be a key discriminator between individuals most negatively affected by retirement and those less negatively affected, intervention might concentrate on developing alternatives or substitutes for family supports for those lacking them, and strengthening family supports for those for whom such structures are available.

It therefore follows that the kind of massive, unwieldly and cost-inefficient interventions implied by much psychiatric epidemiological research up to this point might be replaced by more precise intervention targeting in terms of what kinds of outcomes are to be prevented or treated in what kind of high risk population, identifying patterns of stressors, strains, perceptions, adaptive resources, coping strategies, and personality traits that contribute to the specific impairment. To know, for example, the brute fact that in general, women are more prone to depressive disorders does not suggest any particular viable kind of intervention. Interpreting the results of research in the context of more complex models, both by researchers and by clinically oriented and health service delivery policy concerned consumers, would aid in the precise targeting of intervention efforts.

CURRENT RESEARCH TRENDS: A CRITIQUE

Precise Targeting of High Risk Groups

Unfortunately, precise targeting of high risk populations has been atypical of most field survey research on socio-cultural risk factors. In attempting to summarize some of what is known by researchers concerning the linkages suggested in Figure 12−2, one is struck by the consistent reporting of only two or three variable relationships. It is interesting to note, for example, that when psychiatric epidemiological research findings are summarized, the tendency is to report socio-demographic variable linkages to impairment on a one-to-one level. The Dohrenwends exemplify this stance by painstaking documentation of research that indicates that sex differences are typically found in rates of neurosis (higher for women) and personality disorder (higher for men), and that no consistent sex differences are found in rates of functional psychoses. They also summarize research findings with respect to social class as indicating that higher overall rates of psychiatric disorder are found in the lower classes. The latter relationship holds more for the important subtypes of schizophrenia than for neurosis or manic-depressive psychosis.[16−20]

These conclusive research findings are typical of the literature in that the impact of socio-economic characteristics is analyzed within a one-to-one, unidirectional theoretical framework with little consideration given to the potential interaction between variables themselves, and outcome. Attempting, for example, to sort out racial/ethnic versus social class versus age and sex effects and/or exploring their possible interactional effects on impairment is rare. To be fair, the potential feedback of impairment outcomes on social class has been explored in the social causation versus social selection controversy.[1,16,21] However, there exists a paucity of literature carefully exploring linkages of socio-economic variables to stressors and mediators of specific types in relation to specific impairment outcomes.

Life Change and Life Strain

There is a rapidly proliferating literature on life change as a type of stressor. Although insufficient space in this presentation obviates a thorough description and synthesis of these research efforts, the author has collected the material and is preparing such a synthesis for publication. To date, a large number of articles have been reviewed which link the occurrence of life events with general indicators of psychiatric impairment.[22-45] All of the literature has taken an undifferentiated measure of psychiatric impairment as the dependent variable and has thus limited the relevance of the research to intervention.

Nevertheless, a significant amount of research has been reported which does correlate life event occurrence with specific forms of psychiatric impairment, including anxiety,[34,41,46-52] self-destructive tendencies,[48,49,53,54] depression,[34,41,49,54-58] isolation, mentation problems, delinquency, and aggression,[48] tension, paranoia, and aggression[49], and schizophrenia.[41,54]

Despite their preliminary nature, the major thrust of the findings is apparent: the occurrence of life changes is correlated to the occurrence of a variety of psychiatric impairments, with negative life events generally more strongly related to impairment. Positive events demonstrate mixed relationships to impairment, sometimes being positively linked and sometimes negatively linked.

Again, few efforts have been made in assessing the relative contributions of life change and various socio-economic characteristics with mediators and impairment. Some analyses represent exceptions in that at least socio-economic variables were sometimes controlled and their relative effects on impairment were noted.[32,42,43,58]

Another type of stressor—life strain—has been even less well researched. Though many investigators have examined the influence of life change events on physical and mental illness, the influence of enduring strains (which occur as repeated demands accompanying current roles) has received scant attention. Only very recently have social scientists attempted to measure these chronic stressful situations. Pearlin and Schooler found life strain highly related to the degree of emotional distress individuals reported experiencing in four role areas (marriage, parenting, household economics, and occupation.).[59] Pearlin and Lieberman have presented evidence to support their contention that the impact of major life change events may be largely mediated by the persistent role strains these events impose on individuals.[60] However, since Pearlin and Lieberman examined only a small number of life events, this proposition requires further investigation, as does the role of chronic life strain in psychiatric impairment. A new measure of the latter has been developed by Cohen and Lazarus, and although their instrument, the

"Hassles Scale," has been piloted, it has not yet been used in major survey research.[61]

Subjective Perceptions of Threat

Life event research has recently emphasized that what is more crucial in producing illness behavior may well be the subjective perception of threat by the person experiencing a life event rather than the objective amount of change or strain resulting from the event. This literature has concentrated primarily on (1) the individual's control over the event, and (2) its perceived negative or positive character. It has been demonstrated, for example, that negatively perceived events and/or events beyond the individual's control are more pathogenic than positive events and/or events within the person's control.[63-69]

The author has therefore included perceptions of the degree of threat stemming from a life event or from life strains as major mediator variables in Figure 12−2. If, as the literature intimates, subjective perceptions of threat are prominent mediators between stressors and impairment, one does not have to reach too far in suggesting that subjective perceptions of available adaptive resources may also be significant mediators. Whether an individual feels his or her social supports, financial means, health services, personal qualities and abilities are or are not sufficient to meet the demands of a set of stressors and strains may well determine their pathogenic effect. Although the abundant literature on self esteem certainly bears on the question,[70] to my knowledge this possibility has not been explored in the literature in any direct manner.

Social Support and Health Care Utilization

Figure 12−2 also indicates that the objective availability of adaptive resources is probably another important mediator of change and strain. The literature on social support has become voluminous, implying that social supports are important enough to warrant careful attention to their interaction with the other variables discussed above. Caplan[71] and Cobb[72] have conceptualized social support systems in terms of patterns of information feedback for individuals which validate their expectations concerning themselves and others, thereby maintaining the psychological and physical integrity of the individual over time. The hypothesis furnished in the literature [6,71,73-78] is that social support facilitates coping with crises and adapting to change. Liem and Liem, in some recent work on social network theory, report that it may be the quality rather than the quantity which may be the key to understanding social support as a mechanism of defense against the effects of stressful life events.[79]

The availability of health care services is another noteworthy mediator that has traditionally been examined in terms of its direct impact on impairment, but rarely in terms of how it interacts with other pathogenic variables. Easy or difficult access to public and private clinics, hospitals, and private health care providers may mediate the effect of stressors. The literature suggests that (1) only a minority of individuals with high levels of psychiatric impairment tends to use mental health services, (2) among the users, approximately as many use general health as use specific mental health services, and (3) there are some segments of the population in which under-utilization of services is much greater than in others.[80,81] By contrast, several researchers have reported over-utilization of general health services by clients with psychological problems.[80-83]

In addition, there is a burgeoning and significant literature around the question of what sorts of barriers keep the majority of persons with serious psychiatric problems, particularly those with minority group status, from using health care service facilities.[84-88] Much of this literature does explore the relationship of utilization to various socio-economic variables, but little of it touches on the interaction between health care utilization and the kinds of stressors and mediators detailed in Figure 12−2.

Coping Strategies and Personality Traits

Figure 12−2 depicts two final sets of mediators which would appear to be requisite for an overall assessment and understanding of the social etiology of psychiatric impairment: coping strategies and personality traits. Although there have been few attempts to assess the consequences of individual adoption of varying coping strategies in survey studies, there is flourishing interest in the topic.[59,89] However, while the literature on personality variables seems inexhaustible, the bulk of it has not addressed the life stress and impairment outcome linkage. Rabkin and Streuning write that a variety of personality variables probably affect the life change and illness connection by specifying the conditions under which the connection occurs.[77] The personality set which seems most regularly explored in this vein is what Seeman[90] calls powerlessness,[90] what Schooler and Pearlin call lack of mastery,[77] and what Rotter calls external locus of control.[91] All refer to the tendency of the individual to place responsibility or attribute blame for desirable or undesirable life events on him or herself (internality) or other individuals or circumstances (externality).

Abramowitz, for example, has reported linkages between externality and depressive feelings among college students,[92] and Goss and Morosko[93] have found externality to be related to alcoholism in outpatients.[93] A positive correlation between externality and anxiety has been reported by a number of researchers (e.g., refs. 94, 95). Diagnosed schizophrenics were discovered to be more external than other patients.[96,97] Severity of psychopathology has also been shown to be associated with externality.[98-100] But although linkages of externality to clinically relevant types of psychiatric impairment have been explored, externality as it relates to social antecedents has received little systematic scrutiny. In our own research on four cultural groups, Holmes et al. found that there were no significant differences in locus of control for four cultural groups after the effects of socio-economic variables were controlled and that no significant interaction occurred between socio-economic status and ethnic-cultural group which affects locus of control.[101,102]

AN INTERVENTION IMPLICATION ASSESSMENT PARADIGM

To be frank, the author is much more excited about the *potential* clinical implications of the research trends now emerging than about the implications of what we currently know. Extracting specific clinical inferences from the literature is laborious and difficult in its currently inconsistent and incomplete state and when it primarily deals with relatively undifferentiated forms of psychiatric impairment. A more promising approach to the potential clinical use of general population psychiatric epidemiological research may be represented in the paradigm developed in Figure 12−3. As far as the author has been able to determine, there has been no previous attempt to develop an assessment paradigm of a full range of the practical implications of such research, so the effort attempted in Figure 12−3 should be regarded as tentative and exploratory.

There appear to be two obvious levels at which information generated by psychiatric epidemiology can affect clinical intervention: in terms of how the client and his environment can be altered, and in terms of how the provision of health care service can be altered. Every bit of social scientific information concerning the etiology of psychiatric impairment has potential implications at each level. Figure 12−3 suggests that researchers and practitioners might assess the practical applications of research by simply analyzing the possible consequences of known information concerning socio-economic characteristics, stressors, mediators and all their interactions in terms of how the client and health care services should be modified to maximize effective intervention.

A few additional comments will make the paradigm presented in Figure 12−3 more interpretable and meaningful. Note that research findings are to be assessed in two ways: for the client, and for the health service provider. Since there is no single model of a mentally healthy person which can be formulated

Socio-Cultural Variables	Implications for Intervention			
	Client		Health Service	
	Personal	Environment	Provider Behavior	Provision Structure
I. Socio-Economic Characteristics (SEC) Age Sex Race/Ethnicity Marital Status Social Class Place of Residence Culture SEC Variable Interactions				
II. Stressors (STR) Life Changes Life Strains STR Variable Interactions				
III. SEC X STR Interactions				

IV. Mediators (MED)
 	
Perceptions of Threat
Perceptions of Availability of
   Adaptive Resources
Objective Availability of
   Adaptive Resources
Coping Strategies
Personality Traits
MED Variable Interactions				

V. SEC X MED Interactions				
VI. STR X MED Interactions				
VII. SEC X STR X MED Interactions				

Fig. 12–3. An intervention implication assessment paradigm.

for every form of illness and which would delineate the kind of person who might function effectively in every type of environment, individuals' socio-economic characteristics, patterns of stressors faced, mediators operational in the situation, and the interactions of these components should ideally be taken into account in assessing what a particular client's needs are. Using these guidelines, the mental health practitioner may determine that the kind of personal change or development needed by an Oriental, female, middle-aged, upper middle class client, for example, with relatively stable stressor levels, confident of many available adaptive resources (which objectively exist), and who is suffering from a major depressive disorder might be quite different from behavioral modifications needed by an older, male, white, lower class client with volatile stressor levels, few resources and no self-confidence in his adaptive abilities. The research will undoubtedly prognosticate on what kinds of changes can and should be sought for the client, whether social supports, job, subjective perceptions, etc.

Similarly, research findings can be divided into inferences for effective and desirable individual health care provider behavior and characteristics and for the provision setting in which the practitioner works.

Moreover, the implication for intervention indicated in Figure 12−3 can occur on two levels, either as prevention, or as primary treatment. Drawing directly on the immunological model employed in much public health and general epidemiological literature, psychiatric epidemiological research can be used to identify high risk, under-serviced populations for preventative treatment. As has been consistently argued in this chapter, the more specific and precise the identification, the more potentially effective the intervention. The second level—primary intervention—is obviously the traditional medical model. Here, psychiatric epidemiological research results are probably best crystallized by developing empathic sensibilities in practitioners and health delivery structures to provide help for problems viewed as significant by clients.

For the sake of illustration, we might elaborate a hypothetical, though realistically anticipated, set of research findings and apply the assessment paradigm in the following manner:

A thorough study of young, male, Mexican-American, recently immigrant, lower class residents of a major urban area might well reveal that a disproportionate number of these individuals are experiencing family, work and geographical changes of such significant proportions that the persistent strains associated with the changes are considerable (fear of deportation, absence of key family members, language difficulties, etc.). The study might also demonstrate that the majority of the subjects deal fairly effectively with these changes and stressors by relying heavily on extended family and friendship networks of social support, and that when that social support structure is weak or absent, severe depressive disorders are usually found.

Given these findings, one might entertain the following possible implications for intervention. First, nodal points of intervention for congregations of the target population might be identified: residential areas, rooming houses, day labor pools, treatment facilities with disproportionate numbers of the target group, etc. Then, in terms of both preventative and primary care programs, the specifics of the probable characteristics in need of change in the individual members of the target population could be identified (say, self-esteem or depression), noting that in this particular group, a therapeutic program would have to be carefully devised so as not to violate the relevant cultural values, standards, and expectations concerning proper conduct for, in this case, young males, the role of this type of individual vis à vis his group, and desirable work situations. This strongly suggests that intervention should not be so designed as to make the individual dysfunctional in his own specific cultural/social setting and that general models of desirable outcomes in the treatment of depressive disorders might have to be modified in light of the needs and characteristics of particular target populations.

The research findings might also indicate that particular attention should be given to altering the client's environment in both preventative and primary care programs. Since one aspect of the environment, the presence of social support through friendship networks, was found to be crucial, strengthening social supports could prove therapeutically decisive and would appear to be a more realistic goal than immediate modification of the family or occupational opportunity structure.

With respect to primary care, implications of this research could be assessed both in terms of provider behavior and general structuring of services. With the former, availability and provision of mental health practitioners capable of significant empathy with this particular type of client might be critical. Minimally, that could mean that the therapist should be young, male, conversant in Spanish and knowledgeable in the cultural orientations of this group. Ideally, the practitioner would have sufficient empathy to identify with and understand the client's needs and expectations.

The notion of empathic intervention merits some comment. An increase in empathic abilities would undoubtedly affect clinical processes to the degree that it increases client participation and power in that process. Increased empathy on the part of the practitioner may, in other words, produce a client–professional interaction where more equal bargaining or negotiation could occur, supplying the client with more potential for input and for determining outcome than the more traditional unequal status situation.

In terms of the provision structure, the most effective means of reaching this population would need to be determined. It may well be that the most efficacious structuring of services would probably not lie in the traditional mental health institution with traditional payment and application procedures, but in a group-oriented, neighborhood center.

Undoubtedly, the results of an actual study of such a target group would generate many more specific implications than those we have entertained here. Nevertheless, the author hopes he has shown that not only is some means of formally and consistently assessing practical implications of psychiatric epidemiological research needed, but such means may be developed through the construction of the type of intervention implication assessment paradigm illustrated in this section.

SUMMARY AND CONCLUSIONS

The major thrust of this chapter has been that deriving implications from field studies of the socio-cultural etiology of psychiatric impairment is problematic, but more amenable to solution than has been traditionally assumed. It was argued that a significant gap does indeed exist between research and clinical practice in this area. The origins of that gap were discussed, emphasizing the lack of research instrumentation capable of assessing specific socio-cultural factors and their relationship to specific types of psychiatric impairment. It was suggested that major elements in hindering the development of more viable instrumentation have been the inability of researchers to develop reliable measures of impairment that have a quantifiable relationship to clinically relevant disorder, and the corresponding inability of clinicians to formulate valid, reliable, and measurable diagnostic categories of psychiatric impairment. It was also noted, however, that the current movement toward refinement of reliable diagnostic criteria represented in the DSM-III and in new, closely related field survey instruments provide hope for partially closing the gap.

Another of the author's major contentions was that the full fruits of survey work in psychiatric epidemiology will not be enjoyed until such work originates and is interpreted in the context of multivariate models of the impacts of socio-cultural variables on impairment and which are sensitive to the cumulative, interactive, reciprocal, and multi-leveled nature of those impacts. Such models, though rare in current research, hold the promise of more effective and precise identification of auspicious points of intervention than the typical psychiatric epidemiological research of the past, where relationships of stressors, mediators, and socio-economic variables to impairment generally tend to be reported and interpreted in terms of unidirectional, two- or three-variable models neglecting interactional effects, feedback loops, and the general complexity of the causal sequence in which the particular relationship being analyzed is set. The author is not intimating that every researcher has the responsibility of somehow testing all the components of the theoretical model he has presented in every piece of research, but is suggesting that research would become more practically useful if both researchers and practitioners begin to interpret its results in the context of a similar, complex theoretical model.

An exploratory interpretation and critique of the results of a particular research tradition was then presented and analyzed in terms of the new etiological model. It was shown that both the literature on life change and life strain suggests that the linkages between socio-environmental characteristics, stressors, and impairment is not well understood. What sorts of socio-economic status positions produce what sorts of change and strain, with what consequences for specific types of psychiatric impairment, is not clear, and in the absence of that kind of understanding, the research is not likely to have significant impact on mental health care delivery programs or policy. The selective literature review demonstrated that while there is a wealth of research linking some particular components of major socio-cultural variables to psychiatric impairment, it is seldom interpreted or presented in such a way as to pull together the various elements into an interpretable whole identifying the most promising points of intervention in relation to specific clinical problems in precisely targeted populations. Until that kind of interpretation is available, the practical implications of much psychiatric epidemiological research will remain unexplored.

It was finally argued that even the results of psychiatric epidemiological research embracing multivariate models will not automatically tender practical applications unless researchers and practitioners can develop intervention implication paradigms resembling the experimental example presented in this paper. The author trusts that the approaches he has endeavored to explicate in this chapter, although complex and speculative, could stimulate the stitching of at least some seams along the gap between research and clinical practice.

REFERENCES

1. Faris REL, Dunham HW: Mental Disorders in Urban Areas: An Ecological Study of Schizophrenia and Other Psychoses. Chicago, University of Chicago Press, 1967
2. Srole L, Langner ST, Michael ST, et al: Mental Health in the Metropolis: The Midtown Manhattan Study. New York, McGraw-Hill, 1962
3. Gurin GJ, Veroff J, Feld S: Americans View Their Mental Health: A Nationwide Interview Study. New York, Basic Books, 1960
4. Leighton DC, Harding JS, Macklin DB, et al: The Character of Danger. New York, Basic Books, 1963
5. Dohrenwend BP, Dohrenwend BS: Sex differences and psychiatric disorders. Am J Soc 81:1447–1454, 1976
6. DSM III: DSM-III Draft: Diagnostic and Statistical Manual of Mental Disorders (ed 3). Washington, DC, Am Psychiatric Assoc, 1968
7. Spitzer RT, Endicott J, Robins E: Research Diagnostic Crititeria. New York, Biometrics Research, New York State Psychiatric Institute, 1975
8. Spitzer RT, Endicott J, Robins E: Clinical criteria for psychiatric diagnosis and DSM-III. Am J Psychiatry 132:1187–1192, 1975
9. Spitzer RT, Endicott J, Robins E: Research diagnostic criteria: rationale and reliability. Arch Gen Psychiatry 35:773–782, 1978

10. Feighner JP, Robins E, Guze SB, et al: Diagnostic criteria for use in psychiatric research. Arch Gen Psychiatry 26:57–63, 1972

11. Endicott J, Spitzer RL: A diagnostic interview: The schedule for affective disorders and schizophrenia. Arch Gen Psychiatry 35:837–844, 1978

12. Weissman MM, Myers JK, Hading PS: Psychiatric disorders in a U.S. urban community. Am J Psychiatry 135:459–462, 1978

13. Holmes TH, Rahe RH: The social readjustment rating scale. J Psychosom Res 11:213–218, 1967

14. Rahe RH, Arthur RJ: Life change and illness studies. J Human Stress 4:3–15, 1978

15. Hinkle LE, Wolff HG: Health and the social environment: Experimental investigations, in Leighton AH, Clausen JA, Wilson RN (eds): Explorations in Social Psychiatry. New York, Basic Books, 1957, pp 105–137

16. Dohrenwend BP, Dohrenwend BS: Social Status and Psychological Disorder: A Causal Inquiry. New York, Wiley, 1969

17. Dohrenwend BP, Dohrenwend BS: Sex differences and psychiatric disorders. Paper presented at the VIII World Congress of Sociology, Toronto, Canada, August 19–24, 1974

18. Dohrenwend BP, Dohrenwend BS: Social and cultural influences on psychopathology. Annu Rev Psychol 25:417–452, 1974

19. Dohrenwend BP, Dohrenwend BS: Sex differences and psychiatric disorders. Am J Soc 81:1447–1454, 1976

20. Dohrenwend BP: Sociocultural and social-psychological factors in the genesis of mental disorders. J Health Soc Behav 16:365–392, 1975

21. Grob GN: Introduction in Jarvis, E: Insanity and Idiocy in Massachusetts: Report of the Commission on Lunacy, 1855. Cambridge, Harvard University Press, 1971, pp 1–71

22. Hudgens RW, Robins E, Delong WB: The reporting of recent stress in the lives of psychiatric patients. Br J Psychiatry 117:635–643, 1970

23. Morrison JR, Hudgens RW, Barchha RG: Life events and psychiatric illness: A study of 100 patients and 100 controls. Brit J Psychiat 114:423–432, 1968

24. Dohrenwend BS: Stressful events and psychological symptoms. Paper presented for City College of City University of New York, Conference on Psychosocial Stress Measures: Brief Mental Health Scales in Research and Practice, 1971

25. Dohrenwend BS: Life events as stressors: A methodological inquiry. J Health Soc Behav 14:167–175, 1973

26. Myers JK, Lindenthal JJ, Pepper MP: Life events and psychiatric impairment. J Nerv Ment Dis 152:149–157, 1971

27. Myers JK, Lindenthal JJ, Pepper MP, et al: Life events and mental status: A longitudinal study. J Health Soc Behav 13:398–406, 1972

28. Myers JK, Lindenthal JJ, Pepper MP: Social class, life events and psychiatric symptoms: A longitudinal study, in Dohrenwend BS, Dohrenwend BP (eds): Stressful Life Events: Their Nature and Effects. New York, Wiley, 1974, pp 191–205

29. Coates D, Moyer S, Wellman B: Yorklea study: Symptoms, problems and life events. Can J Public Health 69:471–481

30. Fontana AF, Marcus JL, Noel B, et al: Prehospitalization coping styles of psychiatric patients: The goal directedness of life events. J Nerv Ment Dis 155:311–321, 1972

31. Smith WG: Critical life events and prevention strategies in mental health. Arch Gen Psychiat 25:103–109, 1971

32. Unlenhuth EG, Leipiman RS, Blater MB, et al: Symptom intensity and life stress in the city. Arch Gen Psychiatry 31:759–764, 1974

33. Marx MB, Garrity TF, Bowers FP: The influence of recent life experience on the health of college freshmen. J Psychosom Res 19:89–98, 1975

34. Miller PMc, Ingham JG, Davidson S: Life events, symptoms and social support. J Psychosom Res 20:515–522, 1976

35. Parker DM, Wilsoncraft WE, Olshanek T: The relationship between life change and relative autonomic balance. J Clin Psychol 32:149–153, 1976

36. Payne RL: Recent life changes and the reporting of psychological states. J Psychosom Res 19:99–103, 1976

37. Clum GA: Role of stress in the prognosis of mental illness. J Consult Clin Psychol 44:54–60, 1976

38. Crandell JE, Lehman RE: Relationship of stressful life events to social interest, locus of control and psychological adjustment. J Consult Clin Psychol 45:1208, 1977

39. Garrity TF, Marx MB, Somes GW: Langner's 22 item measure of psychophysiological strain as an intervening variable between life change and health outcome. J Psychosom Res 21:195–199, 1977

40. Marx MB, Garrity TF, Somes GW: The effect of unbalance in life satisfactions and frustrations upon illness. J Psychosom Res 21:423–427, 1977

41. Schwartz CC, Myers JK: Life events and schizophrenia, II: Impact of life events on symptom configuration. Arch Gen Psychiatry 34:1242–1245, 1977

42. Wildman RC, Johnson DR: Life change and Langner's 22 item mental health index: A study and partial replication. J Hlth Soc Behav 18:174–188, 1977

43. Eaton WW: Life events, social supports, and psychiatric symptoms: A re-analysis of the New Haven data. J Health Soc Behav 19:230–234, 1978

44. Mellinger GD, Balter MB, Manheimer DI, et al: Psychiatric distress, life crisis and use of psychotherapeutic medications. Arch Gen Psychiatry 35:1045–1052, 1978

45. Thoits PA: Life Events, Social Integration and Psychological Distress. Unpublished Ph.D. dissertation, Stanford University, 1978

46. Lauer RH: The social readjustment scale and anxiety: A cross-cultural study. J Psychosom Res 17:171–174, 1973

47. Reavley W: The relationship of life events to several aspects of "anxiety." J Psychosom Res 18:421–424, 1973

48. Gersten JL, Langner TS, Eisenberg JG, et al: Child behavior and life events: Undesirable change or change per se?, in Dohrenwend BS, Dohrenwend BP (eds): Stressful Life Events: Their Nature and Effects. New York, Wiley, 1974, pp 159–170

49. Vinokur A, Selzer ML: Desirable versus undesirable life events: Their relationship to stress and mental distress. J Pers Soc Psychol 32:329–337, 1975

50. Ingham JG, Miller P McC: The determinants of illness behavior. J Psychosom Res 20:309–316, 1976

51. Sarason IG, Johnson JH, Siegel JM: Assessing the impact of life changes: Development of the life experiences survey. J Consult Clin Psychol 46:932−946, 1978

52. Roth JT, Hough RL: Anxiety as it is influenced by life change events and internal-external locus of control: A multicultural approach. Paper presented at the Southwestern Sociological Association Meetings, Ft. Worth, Texas, 1979

53. Paykel ES, Prusoff BA, Myers JK: Suicide attempts and recent life events. Arch Gen Psychiatry 32:327−333, 1975

54. Paykel ES: Contribution of life events to causation of psychiatric illness. Psych Med 8:245−253, 1978

55. Brown GW, Sklair F, Harris TO, et al: Life events and psychiatric disorders: I. Some methodological issues. Psychology of Medicine 3:74−87, 1973

56. Paykel ES, Weissman MM: Social adjustment and depression: A longitudinal study. Arch Gen Psychiatry 28:659−663, 1973

57. Paykel ES, Hallowell C, Dressler DM, et al: Treatment of suicide attempts: A descriptive study. Arch Gen Psychiatry 31:487−491, 1974

58. Warheit GJ: Life events, coping, stress, and depressive symptomatology. Am J Psychiat 36:4B, 1979

59. Pearlin LI, Schooler C: The structure of coping. J Hlth Soc Behav 19:2−21, 1978

60. Pearlin LI, Lieberman MA: Social sources of emotional distress, in Simmons R (ed), Research in Community and Mental Health. Greenwich, JAI Press, 1978

61. Cohen BJ, Lazarus RS: The Hassles Scale. Berkeley Stress and Coping Project, The University of California, 1977

62. Lefcourt HM: The function of the illusions of control and freedom. Am Psychol 28;417−425, 1973.

63. Briscoe CW, Smith JB: Psychiatric illness—marital units and divorce. J Nerv Ment Dis 158:440−445, 1974

64. Dohrenwend BP: Problems in defining and sampling the relevant population of stressful life events, in Dohrenwend BS, Dohrenwend BP (eds): Stressful Life Events: Their Nature and Effects. New York, Wiley, 1974, pp 275−310

65. Krantz DS, Glass DC, Snyder ML: Helplessness, stress levels, and the coronary prone behavior pattern. J Exper Soc Psychol 10:284−300, 1974

66. Cassel J: Social science in epidemiology: Psycho-social processes and 'stress' theoretical formulation, in Streuning EL, and Guttentage M (eds): Handbook of Evaluation Research 1:537−549, Beverly Hills, Sage, 1975

67. Cochrane R, Robertson A: Stress in the lives of parasuicides. Soc Psychiatry 10:161−171, 1975

68. Theorell T: Selected illness and somatic factors in relation to two psychosocial stress indices—A prospective study on middle aged construction building workers. J Psychosom Res 20:7−20, 1976

69. Fairbank, DT, Hough RL: Life event classifications and the event-illness relationship. J Human Stress 5:41−47, 1979

70. Wells LE, Maxwell G: Self-esteem: Its conceptualization and measurement. Beverly Hills, Sage, 1976

71. Caplan G: Support Systems and Community Mental Health: Lectures on Concept Development. New York: Behavioral Publications, 1975

72. Cobb S: Social support as a moderator of life stress. Psychosom Med,

38:300−314, 1976

73. Antonovsky A: Conceptual and methodological problems in the study of resistance resources and stressful life events, in Dohrenwend BS, Dohrenwend BP (eds): Stressful Life Events: Their Nature and Effects. New York, Wiley, 1974

74. Myers JK: Life events, social integration and psychiatric symptomatology. J Health Soc Behav 16:421−427, 1975

75. Kaplan BH, Cassel JC: Family and Health: An Epidemiologic Approach. Chapel Hill, Institute for Social Science Research, University of North Carolina, 1975

76. Kaplan BH, Cassel JC, Gore S: Social support and health. Med Care 15:47−58, 1977

77. Rabkin JG, Struening EL: Life events, stress and illness. Science 194:1013−1020, 1976

78. Nuckolls C, Cassel JA, Kaplan B: Psycho-social assets, life crises and the prognosis of pregnancy. Am J Epidemiol 95:431−441, 1972

79. Liem JH, Liem R: Life events, social supports, and physical and psychological well being. Paper presented at the Annual Meeting of the American Psychological Association, 1976

80. Ryan W: Distress in the City. Cleveland, Case Western Reserve University, 1969

81. Andersen R, Francis A, Leon J, et al: Psychologically related illness and health services utilization. Med Care 15:59−73, 1977

82. Tessler R, Mechanic D, Dimond M: The effect of psychological distress on physician utilization: A prospective study. J Health Soc Behav 17:353−364, 1978

83. Mechanic D, Greeley JR: The prevalence of psychological distress and help-seeking in a college student population. Soc Psychiat 11:1−15, 1976

84. McKinley JB: Some approaches and problems in the study of the use of services—An overview. J Health Soc Behav 13:115−152, 1972

85. Aday L, Andersen R: The Development of Indicators of Access to Medical Care. Ann Arbor, Health Administration Press, 1975

86. Wan T, Soifer J: Determinants of physician utilization: A causal analysis. J Health Soc Behav 15:100−112, 1974

87. Wolinsky FD: Health service utilization and attitudes toward health maintenance organizations: A theoretical and methodological discussion. J Health Soc Behav 17:221−236, 1976

88. Greenley JR, Mechanic D: Social selection in seeking help for psychological problems. J Health Soc Behav 17:249−262, 1976

89. Monat A, Lazarus RS: Stress and Coping: An Anthology. New York, Columbia University Press, 1977

90. Seeman M: Empirical alienation studies: An overview, in Geyer RF, Schweitzer DR (eds): Theories of Alienation. Matinus Nijhoff Social Science Division, 1975

91. Lefcourt HM: Locus of Control: Current Trends in Theory and Research. New York, Wiley & Sons, 1976

92. Abramowitz SI: Locus of control and self-reported depression among college

students. Psychol Rep 25:149−150, 1969

93. Goss A, Morosko TE: Relation between a dimension of internal-external control and the MMPI with an alcoholic population. J Consult Clin Psych 34:189−192, 1970

94. Feather NT: Some personality correlates of external control. Aust J Psych 19:253−260, 1967

95. Ray WJ, Katahn M: Relation of anxiety to locus of control. Psych Rep 23:1196, 1968

96. Harrow M, Derrante A: Locus of control in psychiatric patients. J Consult Clin Psych 33:582−589, 1969

97. Cromwell RL, Rosenthal D, Snakow D, Zahn TP: Reaction time, locus of control, choice behavior, and descriptions of parental behavior in schizophrenic and normal subjects. J Pers 29:363−379, 1961

98. Shybut J: Time perspective, internal versus external control and severity of psychological disturbance. J Clin Psych 24:312−315, 1968

99. Smith CE, Pryer MW, Distefano MK: Internal-external and severity of emotional impairment among psychiatric patients. J Clin Psych 27:449−450, 1971

100. Palmer RD: Parental perception and perceived locus of control in psychopathology. J Pers 3:420−431, 1971

101. Holmes M: Ethnicity, socioeconomic status, and internal-external locus of control: A multicultural analysis. Unpublished MA thesis, University of Texas at El Paso, 1976

102. Holmes M, Fairbank DT, and Hough RL: Factor Analysis of the Internal-External Locus of Control Scale in a Multicultural Setting. Working Paper Number 16. El Paso, Life Change and Illness Research Project, The University of Texas at El Paso, 1978

William J. Winslade

13
Ethical Issues

Each of the preceding chapters in this volume deals with specific themes in psychiatric research and practice that give rise to ethical questions. For example, one involves the discovery of better forms of treatment for schizophrenics, requiring experimentation with drugs or other therapies. Experimental treatment may provide benefits to the experimental subjects and eventually to similarly afflicted patients. However, it may also cause harm to the experimental subjects. It is uncertain whether schizophrenic patients have the capacity (competence) to consent to unproven and potentially harmful experimental therapy. Thus one set of ethical issues concerns the relationship between potential benefits and burdens of an experimental treatment; another the rights of patients/subjects to consent to or refuse such treatment. Moreover, these general issues spawn a variety of more specific questions, including the following: How does one decide whether the potential benefits of a drug outweigh the potential risks—at least for the purpose of conducting these needed experimental tests on humans? If the tests are conducted, how should the experimental subjects be selected? What should they be told about the risks and benefits of the tests? Who should supervise the assessment of risk-benefit ratios, selection of subjects, and disclosure of information to them? If the subjects suffer unanticipated harm, such as a new illness, who should provide medical care or compensation to them? These are only a few of the questions that typically arise.

Other examples of ethical issues germane to the links between research and practice cluster around the side-effects of treatments known to be effective. Thus, lithium is the treatment of choice for many persons suffering from manic-depressive psychosis. However, evidence has begun to come in that suggests that lithium may have long-term harmful effects, such as the possibility of renal damage. Do the benefits of the treatment outweigh the harmful side effects? How does one decide this issue? Who should decide? By virtue of what criteria can an ethical decision on this issue be made? These are neither simple nor easy questions to answer.

Still another example can be drawn from the treatment of anorexia nervosa patients. It is well established that anorexics may require long-term treatment combining a variety of therapies including behavior modification, individual psychotherapy, group therapy, occupational therapy, as well as hospitalization and separation from family members. Problems sometimes arise in the course of treatment using behavior modification techniques, such as ''treatment contracts'' that do not allow visitors or phone calls if a patient has not gained the weight specified in the treatment plan. The problem lies in the conditions that violate explicit legal rights. A tension arises between the treatment team's clinical judgment that the deprivation of rights is therapeutically desirable, perhaps necessary, and the realization that this is legally prohibited. Is it ethical to override a patient's legal rights in the name of therapy in the patient's best interests? Apart from questions of legal liability for such conduct, the question of professional responsibility is not easy to resolve in theory or in practice.

These examples touch upon only a few of the many ethical issues that arise in psychiatric research and practice. Other pervasive and difficult ethical problems of contemporary psychiatry have been thoughtfully surveyed by Redlich and Mollica.[1] These issues include the right to be treated or not to be treated; the right to the least restrictive treatment alternatives and the balancing of the individual's right to freedom and society's right to protect itself from possible harm; involuntary commitment and predictions of dangerousness; behavior control through psychopharmacology and psychosurgery; a clarification of whose interests are served in any kind of therapy; privacy and confidentiality weighed against societal needs for information; informed consent in treatment and research, particularly with respect to vulnerable populations; confidentiality in group or couple therapy; and the translation of physician−patient relationship values into governmental policies. Loren Roth et al. has also addressed ethical and legal aspects of psychiatric practice, particularly with respect to competency to consent to treatment.[2] His most recent paper perceptively analyzes the legal and ethical relationships between competency, consent, and treatment in involuntary commitment contexts.[3]

Redlich, Mollica, Roth, and others have begun to identify and systematize the many ethical issues that arise in psychiatric research and practice, and more work must be done in this area. The intent of this essay, however, is to examine two related general themes that will help us to better understand why ethical issues in psychiatry are so complex and so difficult to resolve. First, key aspects of the ethics of professional—client relationships will be examined, with reference to special features of psychiatric research and practice. Second, ethics will be discussed in the context of governmental regulation of research. What is said about forms of regulation applies in general to scientific research and in particular to psychiatric research. The clarification of these two important dimensions is a necessary step toward achieving a more complete and coherent perspective on ethics in psychiatry.

ETHICS IN PROFESSIONAL-CLIENT RELATIONSHIPS

Ethical issues are an integral, though often neglected, part of any analysis of the professional—client relationship. Discussion of ethical issues usually arises in connection with the conduct of the professional, but some attention has recently been given to the responsibilities of clients. Three main topics concerning professionals' conduct are allocation of authority to act, disclosure and consent, and fairness in allocation of benefits and risks to those in need of professional services. The responsibilities of clients include cooperation with and compensation of professionals, and decision-making or its delegation to the professional. In this paper our discussion will be restricted to the ethics of professional conduct; the responsibilities of clients deserve a separate and detailed analysis.

Cultural traditions, personal belief systems, political practices, and legal rules have created a complex process resulting in the allocation of substantial authority to professionals. In twentieth century America, professionals (and especially physicians) have been granted extraordinary powers to shape the personal and collective values of their clients. For example, physicians have exercised considerable discretion in deciding about withholding or withdrawing life support from terminally ill or comatose patients, deciding whether or not to perform surgery on children with conditions such as spina bifida, recommending and greatly influencing the choices of therapies of cancer patients, and deciding whether or not a person with a mental disorder should be involuntarily hospitalized. These decisions have a significant impact upon the lives and families of patients. How and why this process occurred is a rich subject for sociological and historical analysis that lies beyond the scope of this paper.[4]

Ethical issues arise because allocation of authority inevitably creates a risk of abuse and exploitation. Unless the exercise of authority is subject to criticism and review, even benevolent motives may produce authoritarian consequences. It is not uncommon to learn after the fact that persons with authority to act in secret e.g., the CIA or the FBI, have abused their power. Similarly, persons whose exercise of authority is rarely public, such as some staffs of mental hospitals, may intentionally exploit or unintentionally harm their clients.[5] Individual psychiatrists cloaked with the power and authority of transference may also exploit their patients. The recent controversy about sexual contacts between therapists and patients illustrates the potential for abuse. I make no claims about the frequency of abuse; I want only to stress the potential for abuse that accompanies the allocation of substantial authority to professionals.[6]

A second generally recognized ethical dimension of professional-client relationships concerns disclosure and consent. Professionals are obligated to disclose to their clients the nature of the services they offer and the skills they possess. After helping potential clients to identify their problems, a professional has a duty to make a recommendation about the risks and benefits of alternative solutions. Of course, a professional may advise a client as to a preferred alternative and what he or she can specifically offer a client. An orthopedist may advise a patient with a broken bone of the risks and benefits of traction in contrast to surgery and may recommend one or the other. But it is up to the patient—if a competent adult—to consent to or refuse either or both proposed forms of treatment. The professional must disclose enough relevant information to enable the client to make a rational choice; the client has the right and duty to consent or refuse to consent. Of course the client may waive the right to receive certain information and may allocate much decision-making authority to a professional to act as his or her agent.[7]

Ethical issues typically arise in disclosure and consent situations when professionals fail to disclose enough or in a manner appropriate to a client's needs. For example, professionals who do not disclose relevant information may fail to respect the moral autonomy of their clients. Even if a professional sincerely believes it is in the best interest of the client not to know something risky or unpleasant, unless the authority not to disclose has been specifically acknowledged, the professional may be violating the rights of a client. This is a typical claim in many medical malpractice cases. Professionals sometimes underestimate their clients' need and sometimes disregard their right to know.

A third area that raises ethical questions has to do with whether services provided are fairly distributed to those in need or whether risks that are taken are inappropriately placed upon certain populations. Questions of social justice—allocation of benefits and burdens—are persistently raised about the activities of professionals. Whether the institutionalized mentally disabled receive less adequate care than private psychiatric patients, and whether institutionalized patients are subjected to greater risks because of their more frequent participation in psychiatric research, are some examples of this controversy.[5]

Although ethical issues in psychiatric research and practice are not essentially different from other areas of professional activity, there are special factors that contribute to the sensitivity about ethics in psychiatry. Psychiatrists often deal with problems that involve a person's most intimate feelings, beliefs, or conduct. This may include fantasies or behavior that violates accepted legal or moral standards. Or it may concern information that is embarrassing to the patient. The precautions taken to protect the privacy of patients—even that they are psychiatric patients—reflect the fact that psychiatrists' inquiries are potentially intrusive because they are concerned with intimate knowledge. To obtain and maintain patients' trust, psychiatrists must provide confidentiality in treatment and research settings.[8]

Another respect in which psychiatry is potentially intrusive is in the forms of treatment. Psychiatric treatment often is intended to affect significant aspects of a patient's personality. Some forms of treatment—psychosurgery and other organic therapies—may cause major alterations in a person's emotional life. Drugs may have not only a short-term but also a long-term impact on a patient. Even the "talking therapies" may probe and influence extremely sensitive dimensions of personality. Professionals who routinely deal with these phenomena may lose sight of the fact that psychiatric treatment is very traumatic for patients. This is particularly true because at the time treatment is needed, patients are unusually vulnerable to being harmed because they are in volatile emotional states.

The intimacy and vulnerability of psychiatric situations, and the intrusiveness of patient treatment, underlie the significance of transference phenomena in psychiatric treatment. Psychiatrists acquire, by virtue of their special knowledge and power, a de facto authority and influence over their patients' emotional lives. Thus they have a special duty to exercise this authority and influence with great caution and sensitivity.

Another special feature of the psychiatric context is that many patients suffer to some degree from temporary or permanent disabilities that affect their competence. Emotional or organic problems may prevent a patient from comprehending or appreciating a psychiatrist's disclosure. Psychiatrists may also reasonably believe that certain disclosures to an emotionally disturbed patient may be detrimental to treatment at a particular time. It is sometimes presumed that psychiatric patients are incompetent, and patients who have learned to appear helpless reinforce this presumption. The appearance or presumption of incompetence further encourages psychiatrists to override the client's ideas about what is best for him or her.

The current controversy about ethical issues in psychiatry has been enlivened by critics from within as well as outside the profession. Szasz, Laing and their followers have for years proliferated a polemic against psychiatric practice. Their radical critique, though excessive, has put some psychiatrists on the defensive or made those who dismiss radical critics lightly seem arrogant. External critics—former patients, legal critics, and government officials, as well as a sceptical public (fed by movie-land and popular novel images of psychiatry)—have called into question the authority, effectiveness and integrity of psychiatric research and practice.

ETHICS AND GOVERNMENT REGULATION OF PSYCHIATRIC RESEARCH

Psychiatric practice can generally be divided into two types: institutional and private. For a variety of reasons, including size, institutional practice tends to generate the greatest amount of research. As a result, government regulation is more pronounced in public institutions. These institutions, usually funded (or under-funded) with public moneys, also have a disproportionate number of the poor and minorities among their patient population. As a result, the poor and minorities are more often subjects of psychiatric research. Because of this, there is greater concern about the assessment of risks and benefits, and the need for close regulation of these facilities is more fully expressed. Since private hospital patients have more options open to them, it is felt that they are in a better position either to protect themselves or to be protected by their families with respect to participation in research.

It is clear that much more information is needed. Before ethical and legal issues in psychiatric research and practice can be fruitfully analyzed, we need to know more about actual research practices as they relate to ethical issues. Unfortunately, there has been little empirical research directed toward assessing these questions. Within the larger medical community some research on this topic has been conducted. As well, certain notorious cases have created significant public and professional concern: the Jewish Chronic Disease Hospital case, the Tuskegee Syphilis Study, and the Willowbrook Study, among others, gave rise to the legislation that created the National Commission for the Protection of Human Subjects of Biomedical and Behavioral Research. Although these dramatic instances of alleged human subject research abuses provoked concern and action, it is still the case that apart from some valuable studies authorized by the Commission, very little information exists about the extent to which scientific investigators do or do not exploit, abuse, or mislead human subjects in nontherapeutic or therapeutic research. Even Beecher's famous article on "Ethics and Clinical Research" alerts us only through brief and nonsystematic accounts of possible abuses.[9] Despite this lack of documented evidence of systematic or substantial abuse (except in what may be isolated cases), concern about vulnerable populations has spawned a proliferation of ethical debates, legal regulations, and public discussions.

The case that is made for greater regulation of research rests largely upon isolated reports rather than discovery of systematic abuses. However, none of these cases has involved psychiatric research. Thus, official and regulatory concern with psychiatric subjects does not result from tales of abuse, but from the mere fact of patients' vulnerability and of the potential for abuse. The concern derives from abstract notions rather than pragmatic need. Not having to counter specific abuses, there may be a tendency in providing regulation to try to prevent all possible abuses without sufficient consideration of the disadvantages as well as the advantages of stringent regulation.

The National Commission, during its four-year existence (1974 – 1978) studied and made recommendations concerning psychiatric research and practice involving psychosurgery, and psychiatric research involving those institutionalized as mentally infirm. These recommendations were made in the absence of sufficient empirical knowledge about the need for regulation, although they were made in the light of hearings, site visits, analytical papers, and some incompletely and inadequately analyzed empirical research. Subsequently, DHEW issued proposed regulations (going substantially beyond the recommendations of the National Commission) that would significantly restrict psychiatric research. The most striking feature of the proposed DHEW regulations is the requirement for consent monitors and patient advocates in certain situations where psychiatric patient/subjects are at special risks.[5]

Increased legal regulations may or may not be warranted. That is, despite protests from the research community that they do not exploit patient/subjects, it may be that consistent abuses do occur. It may also be that researchers are more sensitive to the ethical issues than their critics claim or than even the researchers themselves realize. It is clear, however, that at least minimal regulation is needed to protect human subjects from actual and potential abuse by investigators, by ensuring that even competent subjects who agree to participate have been given adequate information and have exercised free choice. Some potential subjects may fail to appreciate, or may disregard, the seriousness of risks to which they may be subjected. In such cases, regulation is needed to set limits for permissible participation, in order to protect potential subjects from themselves. But precisely what regulations are needed in psychiatric research is not yet clear.

Not only human subjects but also investigators benefit from regulation. First, regulations requiring evidence of the informed consent of experimental subjects protect investigators from tort liability for unconsented infringement on a person's right to personal integrity. By requiring sufficient documentation, the government protects investigators from unwarranted future complaints. Second, the regulations remind scientists that other values, e.g., personal integrity, and freedom of choice, may come into conflict with the values of scientific knowledge, and that one must proceed cautiously in the face of such potential conflict.

Several political factors have influenced recent developments regarding research with human subjects, including, but not limited to, psychiatry. First, the money spent on medical research has increased enormously in the past three decades.[10,11] Much of this financial support has come from government rather than private sources, and politicians have become involved in its dispensation. The amount of political intervention is not necessarily tied to the amount of allocated funds, but there is clearly increased vulnerability to external controls and regulation as the amounts increase. Especially when scandalous practices are exposed, the government typically responds by passing legislation designed to prevent future abuses. For example, the legislation that established the National Commission was given great impetus by the disclosure of the Tuskegee Syphilis Study in which the investigators, after learning that penicillin could cure venereal disease, nevertheless allowed the disease to run its course for the sake of the experiment.

A second political reality is that licensed professionals—physicians, attorneys, engineers, architects, etc.—are subject to much greater public scrutiny than in the past. Not only are the government and the consumers seeking to protect individuals from receiving inadequate professional services, but professionals through their professional organizations have begun to reexamine professional standards of conduct and competence. The result is that professional accountability has become a significant background factor in medical experimentation. Because the articulation of professional standards by professionals themselves has long been neglected, others, primarily government agencies and consumer groups, have sought to establish and impose such standards.[12]

FORMS OF REGULATION OF SCIENTIFIC RESEARCH

Ethics

Person-Oriented versus Benefit-Oriented Morality. The most fundamental ethical tension arises between two types of moralities germane to research with human subjects: a benefit-oriented versus a person-oriented morality. This distinction, articulated in Paul Ramsey's "The Patient as a Person," is crucial to an understanding of the ethics of human experimentation.[13,14] A benefit-oriented ethics appeals to the preponderance of benefits over costs as a justification for medical experimentation. A person-oriented ethics is grounded upon the fundamental rights of persons to be respected. For example, testing a new vaccine on soldiers might be very beneficial to society, but to do so without informing them of the risks or giving them an opportunity to refuse to participate would be moral exploitation.

These two ethical orientations need not be in conflict, but they do represent positions that appeal to different fundamental values. A benefit-oriented ethics would stress the importance of a favorable risk/benefit ratio as a primary justification for medical experimentation; a person-oriented ethics relies more heavily on protection of personal autonomy by means of strict adherence to informed consent requirements. Those who favor a benefit-oriented ethics tend to dismiss the value of informed consent by questioning its validity, that is, whether consent can ever be adequately informed or sufficiently free. They emphasize instead the potential benefits of the research, in assessing whether the risk to human subjects is justifiable. Conversely, those who favor a person-oriented ethics challenge the reliability of predictions of risk/benefit assessments; they prefer to take extra precautions to ensure that the subjects are competent, informed, comprehending, and free. Of course both aspects are relevant to any proposed experiment, but the tension between these two, sometimes conflicting, ethical orientations partly explains the hesitation many persons have about the human experimentation enterprise.

Ethical Codes.   Several ethical codes, such as the Nuremberg, Geneva, and the Helsinki Codes, have been formulated to strike a proper balance between the social benefits of scientific knowledge and the personal rights of experimental subjects. The 1947 Nuremberg Code places great emphasis on informed consent and protection of experimental subjects, perhaps in reaction to the Nazi abuses. The Helsinki Code, as revised in 1975, presents a more evenly balanced approach toward the interests of society in increasing knowledge and the interests of subjects in protection from exploitation. However, these ethical codes are only guidelines, not strict standards that control scientific investigators.

An international consensus establishing enforceable international standards has been slow to develop. It is to be hoped that the international medical research community in cooperation with other professionals will take the lead in translating advisory documents like the Helsinki Code into more specific and enforceable ethical and legal instruments. It is difficult to be optimistic about the international political environment becoming sufficiently stable for this to occur through intergovernmental agreements alone. But professionals in law, medicine, and related fields could initiate activity that would lead to the adoption of appropriate guidelines and limits for human subject research.

Law

Legal uncertainties arise because of the lack of effective international consensus on regulation of human experimentation; the absence of sufficient case law concerning medical inquiry in humans; scanty statutory guidelines; and cumbersome and superficial administrative regulations. Despite considerable rhetoric in the legal community, it is likely that the law will follow rather than lead the development of social policy in this area. But the scientific community's misconceptions about the current state of the law do add to the growing confusion about standards of practice required by law.

The greatest amount of legal regulation over experimentation with human subjects in the United States is imposed by administrative agencies i.e. Department of Health, Education and Welfare; National Institutes of Health; National Institute of Mental Health; and Public Health Service, over investigators and institutions receiving federal research funds. Prior to the awarding of federal grants, scientific protocols for research involving human subjects must be reviewed by an Institutional Review Board of the investigator's institution and by the appropriate federal agency. This administrative review process assesses the written research proposal with respect to potential benefits and risks, and the adequacy of informed consent documents. The review process concentrates primarily on the design and documentation of human experimentation rather than on the actual conduct of the research. Although in recent years there has been much talk about the monitoring of medical research on humans, very little has been done to study empirically the extent to which human subjects are in fact subjected to undisclosed or unwarranted risks. The administrative regulations at least provide a certain amount of self-consciousness about, and impose minimum standards for, evaluation of risks, benefits, and adequacy of informed consent.[15] Unfortunately, however, many investigators view the administrative review process largely as a bureaucratic burden, rather than as a meaningful attempt to protect human subjects.

SELF-DETERMINATION AND PATERNALISM: PRINCIPLES IN DYNAMIC TENSION

Until the last 25 years, scientists were largely self-regulating, but during these past 25 years, there has been a shift from self-determination to paternalism. However, it is helpful to view it as a shift from self-regulation by scientists to paternalism by government (what may be called bureaucratic paternalism) toward scientists and to a great extent toward research subjects as well. The relevance of paternalism and self-determination as limiting principles toward both scientists and research subjects has not been sufficiently appreciated and discussed in the current literature.

Until recently, it was assumed that each individual scientist would maintain high standards of personal and professional integrity. In rare cases a scientist's employer or professional society might need to intervene to prevent exploitation or overreaching. For the most part, however, the scientific community (like other professional groups) did not give much attention to formulating or enforcing ethical or legal principles for research on human subjects.

It was taken for granted that each scientist, subject to normal peer pressures to produce rigorous research and to survive critical review in professional journals, would develop scientifically sound and ethically permissible research designs. If doubt were to arise, a scientist would be expected to consult with more experienced colleagues. However, in recent years, the instances of exploitation and abuse mentioned earlier, as well as increasing public distrust of professionals, have created governmental concern that at least some scientists can not be trusted to provide proper self-regulation. Furthermore, because there had been no tradition of systematic review of the ethics of research protocols, scientists could produce no convincing evidence to demonstrate how frequently (or infrequently) actual or potential abuse of human subjects was a problem. Despite sincere, as well as self-righteous, protests from the scientific community, the politicians and governmental agencies moved in with regulations, reporting requirements and, more recently, institutional review boards. It is clear that institutional review boards are already deeply entrenched as part of governmental as well as university bureaucracy. Although their power and influence varies from institution to institution, the trend is toward assigning them ever greater responsibilities for regulation of research.

One of the consequences of the growth of administrative regulation of medical research is bureaucratic paternalism. For our present purposes, paternalism refers to a situation in which someone other than the person who is the actor—a parent for a child, a government agency for a citizen, a psychiatrist for a patient—is authorized to determine what is in the person's best interest and to control the person's choices or conduct accordingly. Bureaucratic paternalism occurs when government agencies, institutional review boards, or other review bodies rather than investigators establish regulations that define procedures and set limits to scientific research. The most familiar form this paternalism takes is in specifying risk-benefit ratios and informed consent requirements. In both cases, the administrative review process is employed to determine the scientific and ethical appropriateness of a particular research protocol. Although this process is said to be for the protection of human subjects, its actual direct effect is to impose paternalistic limitations on researchers. The administrative review process protects the research subject only indirectly, if at all, for the review is made only of the protocols submitted by scientists to funding agencies, not of the actual research. Administrative approval, which is required prior to receiving funds from federal agencies, is a form of purse-string paternalism not unlike a parent's withholding of money to manipulate children.

An alternative to bureaucratic paternalism would be to impose fewer restrictions on scientific investigators in the design and conduct of their research but to carefully monitor for exploitation and abuse. In addition, investigators could be held personally responsible for their conduct. That is, sanctions could be imposed by professional licensing and regulatory organizations, or civil and criminal liability might be imposed.[16] Many scientists might initially recoil at this suggestion because of a concern that this would open the litigation floodgates. There may be occasional cases that would and should be subject to a lawsuit. But the likelihood of frequent or disruptive punitive legal action is far less certain than the inevitable and relentless expansion of bureaucratic regulation. Monitoring of the conduct of scientists and the consequences of human subject research is needed to find out the extent to which research subjects are exposed to, or suffer harm. Current attempts to build monitoring into the administrative review process are more rhetoric than reality. They serve only as window dressing for business as usual.

Although there has been a shift from self-regulation to paternalistic regulation of scientists, it may seem that a shift from paternalism to self-determination has occurred toward research subjects—at least in theory. This shift is symbolized, but not necessarily made real, by the rigorous informed consent requirements now attached to human subject research. It is commonly said that the purpose of informed consent requirements is to protect the autonomy, self-determination and personal rights of research subjects.

Prior to the rise of the informed consent doctrine, participants in human subject research were typically children, prisoners and hospital patients. It was assumed that persons responsible for the custody and care of such persons would make benevolent, but nonetheless paternalistic, decisions on behalf of such subjects. As pointed out earlier, actual and potential exploitation and abuse occurred under this system. As a result, the administrative review process now limits the eligibility of certain classes of persons to participate in human subject research. Thus, fetuses, prisoners, children, and the mentally disabled are eligible as research subjects only under strict limitations, if at all. The proposed federal regulations requiring consent monitors and patient advocates in many areas of psychiatric research illustrate this trend. In addition, potential research subjects who are eligible must be informed, competent, comprehending, and free to consent or to refuse to participate. To the extent that informed consent requirements are rigorously enforced, the pool of research subjects will be diminished still more. The result is that informed consent requirements are in effect a form of bureaucratic paternalism toward potential research subjects. It may be desirable that paternalism be exercised in this area to protect vulnerable populations against exploitation or abuse, but it should be recognized that the official rationale for informed consent requirements—that is, to protect individual autonomy—does not tell the whole story, and is even misleading. The requirements have been established in part to protect willing subjects from making their own possibly unwise decisions.

The greatest danger of bureaucratic paternalism is that it will transform the dynamic tension between self-determination and paternalism into administrative rigidity. Scientists must be permitted to pursue research without the burden of punitive regulations. Human subjects must be protected from abuse and from harm. Yet most regulation of human experimentation, at least in the United States, has been only indirectly related to protecting human subjects. Instead, the emphasis has been on technical reviews of protocol statements rather than on substantive investigation of what actually happens to the people participating in the experiments in question. Even less attention has been given to providing insurance for medical care and compensation for those who are accidentally injured. Thus bureaucratic paternalism fails to strike a proper balance between self-determination and paternalism. Scientists should be held accountable for their conduct, not badgered by bureaucrats. Human subjects must be directly protected, not become merely the indirect and remote beneficiaries of administrative regulations. Both scientists and experimental subjects must be treated with the respect due to them as rational and free agents capable of self-determination subject to minimal and reasonable paternalistic controls. To achieve this goal, the current trend toward the quagmire of bureaucratic paternalism must be reversed.

REFERENCES

1. Redlich F, Mollica R: Overview: Ethical issues in comtemporary psychiatry. Am J Psychiatry 134:125−136, 1976
2. Roth L, Meisel A, Lidz C: Tests of competency to consent to treatment. Am J Psychiatry 134:279−284, 1977
3. Roth L: A commitment law for patients, doctors and lawyers. Am J of Psychiatry 136:1121−1127, 1979
4. Collins R: The Credential Society: A Historical Sociology of Education and Stratification, New York, Academic Press, 1979
5. National Commission for the Protection of Human Subjects. Report and recommendations: Research involving those institutionalized as mentally infirm, DHEW, 1978, pp 59−61; and *Appendix*
6. Riskin L: Sexual relations between psychotherapists and their patients: Toward research or restraint. Calif Law Rev 67:1000−1027, 1979
7. Hagman D: The medical patient's right to know: Report on a medical-legal-ethical study. UCLA Law Rev 17:757−816, 1970
8. Winslade WJ: Confidentiality, in Reich W (ed): Encyclopedia of Bioethics. New York, Macmillan, 1979, pp 1443−1447

9. Beecher HK: Ethics and clinical research. New Engl J Med 274:1354—1360, 1966

10. Price D: Endless frontier or bureaucratic morass? Daedalus, Limits of Scientific Inquiry 12:75—92, 1978

11. Brooks H: The problem of research priorities. Daedalus, Limits of Scientific Inquiry 12:171—190, 1978

12. Nelkin D: Threats and promises: Negotiating the control of research. Daedalus, Limits of Scientific Inquiry 12:191—210, 1978

13. Ramsey P: The Patient as a Person. New Haven, Yale University Press, 1970

14. Winslade W: A critical study of Paul Ramsey's "The Patient as a Person." Institute on Human Values in Medicine, Report of Fellows 1973—74, Philadelphia, 1974

15. Gray B, Cooke R, Tannenbaum A: Research involving human subjects. Science 201:1094—1101, 1978

16. Human Experimentation, Chapter 1.3, Section 24170 ff., Division 20, Health and Safety Code, State of California, 1978

INDEX